LOSE WEIGHT, FEEL GOOD

THE BEST STEPS TO TAKE

GANIHU ONYEBUASHI

© **Copyright 2022 - All rights reserved.**

The content contained within this book may not be reproduced, duplicated, or transmitted without direct written permission from the author or the publisher.

Under no circumstances will any blame or legal responsibility be held against the publisher, or author, for any damages, reparation, or monetary loss due to the information contained within this book, either directly or indirectly.

Legal Notice:

This book is copyright protected. It is only for personal use. You cannot amend, distribute, sell, use, quote, or paraphrase any part, or the content within this book, without the author or publisher's permission.

Disclaimer Notice:

Please note that the information contained within this document is for educational and entertainment purposes only. All effort has been executed to present accurate, up-to-date, reliable, complete information. No warranties of any kind are declared or implied. Readers acknowledge that the author is not rendering legal, financial, medical, or professional advice. The content within this book has been derived from various sources. Please consult a licensed professional before attempting any techniques outlined in this book.

By reading this document, the reader agrees that under no circumstances is the author responsible for any losses, direct or indirect, that are incurred due to the use of the information in this document, including, but not limited to, errors, omissions, or inaccuracies.

This book is dedicated to my wife, Amaka Onyebuashi and my two children, Keneolisa and Kobimdi Onyebuashi for their support in writing this book. I love you all

CONTENTS

Introduction	9
1. THE BENEFITS OF A HEALTHY BODY	13
Benefits of a healthy lifestyle	14
Effects of bad lifestyle	19
2. THE TOP 10 NATURAL WAYS TO TONE DOWN YOUR BODY	29
1. Eat small meals	29
2. Exercise	32
3. Drink more water	44
4. Consume foods high in fiber.	49
5. Watch your daily intake of salt	54
6. Have a crunchy snack daily to satisfy your need for something creaky	58
7. Consume less red meat and dairy products	58
8. Eat more whole grains	59
9. Be Realistic	61
10. Get enough sleep	62
3. HEALTH BENEFITS OF A BALANCED DIET	67
How much protein, fat, and carbohydrates should I have?	70
Micronutrients	76
4. WEEKLY MENU PLAN FOR WEIGHT LOSS	83
How to make a weight-loss meal plan	84
Breakfast Recipes	85
Lunch Recipes	91
Dinner	97

Snacks	108
What the research says	113
5. BODY FAT PERCENTAGE AND IDEAL WEIGHT CHART, BMI CALCULATOR	117
Overweight, Obesity, and Body Fat	117
How Much Body Fat Percentage Is Too Much?	120
What Should You Do If You Fall Outside of Those Ranges?	121
Who wouldn't benefit from using a BMI calculator?	124
Guideline for weight and height	126
6. WHAT IS CHOLESTEROL? WAYS TO LOWER YOUR CHOLESTEROL	129
The Facts	129
Essential nutrients that help improve cholesterol levels	133
7. HEALTH BENEFITS OF YOGA	139
How does Yoga Help With Weight Loss?	143
When it comes to losing weight, how often should you practice yoga?	146
Poses to practice at home	147
8. SUPERFOODS TO AVOID FOR WEIGHT LOSS	155
SuperFoods for Weight Loss	162
9. THINGS TO AVOID WHILE TRYING TO LOSE WEIGHT	173
Here are 15 common weight-loss blunders that people make	173
Losing weight too fast	192
10. CALORIES IN FOOD AND CALORIE	195
Calorie information	196

11. CALORIE DEFICIT   207
    The Daily Percentage Value (DV%)   218

12. GETTING TO AND MAINTAINING   221
    YOUR IDEAL WEIGHT
    11 Things To Know Before You Start   222
    Losing Weight

    RECIPES FOR CALORIE DEFICIT   225

    Conclusion   249
    Glossary   257
    Bibliography   261

INTRODUCTION

The health world changes drastically yearly. Food trends that are new for one year are old news the next, and everyone is jumping on the latest trend to lose weight. From apple cider vinegar to veganism, these diet plans seem never to die out. Yet some people struggle with their weight year in and year out with little success except for a few pounds of loss and then back to the same old weight. Many others turn to fad diets that are in and out of style every year in hopes of changing their bodies and weight once and for all. However, some people have been on diets all their life with little success because they don't seem to find a food diet that works for them.

The answer is clear; you need to change your core life diet. It may be frustrating that the latest trend or diet does not work for you, but remember, this is not your fault. The problem is the diet itself; it does not appeal to your body or fit your lifestyle. Many diets do not fit into one simple category, and the realization of this makes it difficult to find a diet that works.

You can change things in your life to make a more favorable environment for losing weight. How much is written in the stars, how much our body can tolerate, and how many calories we need to eat all play a role in how much we will lose when trying to lose weight. The key is knowing these things about yourself before beginning any diet and making the most out of them.

You can still lose weight. To make the process easier for you, all it takes is a little thought and effort.

This book entails a list of the things you should change to lose weight feeling better physically and mentally. It's all about changing your lifestyle to be healthier when it comes to losing weight. It does not just change you physically but mentally as well.

The first step in losing weight is the most difficult. You have to see the fact that you need to change. Understanding the fundamentals of changing your life to be healthier can make the process at least a little less difficult.

Don't give up. You cannot change your life or your habits by yourself; this is a process that will take time and effort. It may be easier to go back to the old habit of unhealthy eating and gain the weight back than it is to change it, but the results will be worth it in the long run.

Until you have lost weight, there are things you have to change to maintain that weight loss when you've got it down. It's nice to see results, but eating well and exercising regularly is important. These are healthy habits too, so it's not like you're giving up all good things by changing to lose weight.

This book includes a practical guide that walks you through the process of losing weight, along with a series of tips on how to keep that weight off. Losing weight is never easy, but having a plan and sticking with it will make the process easier for you.

There is a definite process to losing weight. It's not a quick process, but every journey begins with a single step. The same is true of your weight loss journey. Some days will be harder than others, but you need to keep at it if you want to lose weight in the long run.

You should do some things every day and some days of the week to make your weight loss easier and more effective if they are done right. Some things will be easier than others; don't think you have to do everything all at once or that when one thing doesn't work for you, there is nothing else that could work for you. It may take time, but with a little bit of time and effort, you can change the way you look and feel.

There are many things to consider when starting a weight loss journey. This book will help you think about the things to consider to plan the right path for yourself.

1

THE BENEFITS OF A HEALTHY BODY

It is important to maintain a healthy weight for many reasons. This includes your physical appearance and the medical benefits of having a lower BMI. You should also know that people with a healthy body weight tend to live longer.

Although most people associate a healthy body weight with a number on the scale, it is not always accurate. After all, your weight can fluctuate throughout the day, especially if you are dehydrated and don't consider variables such as your age or height. Experts agree that there are certain ways to decrease your weight by using natural methods. You'll be able to tell if you're not feeling well. You may feel "off," noticing that you're tired, your digestive system isn't working as well as it should, and you're catching colds more frequently than usual. You may be unable to concentrate and feel anxious or depressed as a result. If this is the case, you may consider losing weight to improve your physical and mental health.

It's crucial to live a healthy lifestyle by doing things that make you happy and feel good.

It may be enough for one person to walk a mile five times a week, eat fast food once a week, and spend virtual or in-person time with loved ones every other day. Five miles per week, fast food once per week, and virtual or in-person time with loved ones every other day may be sufficient for one person.

Neither of these options is superior to the other. Both are ideal for that individual. You get to choose how you want to live a healthy lifestyle, whether eating a couple of steamed vegetables every night or sleeping 12 hours a day.

BENEFITS OF A HEALTHY LIFESTYLE

Changes in lifestyle can benefit your body, mind, wallet, and even the environment.

Prevents disease

Healthy habits can help you avoid various diseases, including diseases that run in your families, such as diabetes and heart disease. Research shows that eating a well-balanced diet, exercising regularly, making smart lifestyle choices, and getting regular checkups at the doctor's office can help your body remain in top condition throughout your life span.

Reduces stress

Another benefit of a healthy lifestyle is reducing stress on your body. Stress is known to cause high blood pressure and other cardiovascular problems and an increased risk of stroke and heart attack.

When you do not have high blood pressure or diabetes symptoms, it is difficult to receive medical help or treatments that could help with these conditions. Physical health problems are synonymous with physical disabilities that prevent us from doing things we want in life.

Enhances your overall health

A healthy lifestyle can help complement the health of your organs and other systems in your body. Staying in good shape can benefit your eyesight as well as your mental and physical health.

Consuming the right kinds of food, exercising regularly, and getting a good night's sleep can help keep your organs and other bodily systems in top condition.

You will enjoy your days more than if you aren't doing these things regularly with proper care.

Increases your life expectancy

As mentioned above, people in good physical shape tend to live longer than individuals who do not take care of their bodies well. Maintaining a healthy lifestyle can help to prevent obesity-related diseases like heart disease and cancer. These diseases are known for causing premature death in otherwise healthy individuals.

When you live longer, you have more opportunities to achieve important personal goals, such as getting married or starting a family. You will also spend more time with your loved ones and make lifetime memories.

Improves your mood

While maintaining a healthy physical state can help you feel more energized and less stressed, it does not ensure that you will always feel great. It all depends on how you currently treat yourself and others around you. It is easier to laugh, play, explore, and make new friends in better physical shape. This can lead to a happier emotional experience because of the great new experiences of being healthy and fit.

Reduces chronic pain

Many people believe that exercise is always a great way to rid themselves of joint and muscle pain, but it is not the only way. You can also reduce chronic pain by pursuing a healthy lifestyle. It will be easier for you to exercise if you are in good physical shape, which has been shown to help relieve painful symptoms caused by diseases like arthritis and fibromyalgia.

It might be easy to focus on the health benefits of being in good physical shape, but there are also financial benefits of living this type of lifestyle.

Saves money

Often, people are concerned that a healthy lifestyle will cost them more money. Although this may be the case if you frequently go out to eat at expensive restaurants or buy lots of items from pricey stores, there are also many ways to save money when you are in good physical shape. For example, you could start walking to work instead of driving your car and take advantage of free or low-cost local events and entertainment options in your area.

If you do not have any chronic health problems, the only medical costs that would concern you would be checkups with a doctor every few years and prescriptions for occasional colds or other illnesses.

Gives peace of mind

If you have children, a healthy lifestyle can help them stay in their best shape and provide them with more opportunities to excel in school or succeed at competitive sports. If you are a parent, you will feel happy knowing that you are taking good care of your children and helping them achieve their dreams.

In addition to the physical health benefits, living a healthy lifestyle also provides peace of mind because it allows you to stop worrying about physical disabilities. What being unhealthy might do to your life choices, such as being able to travel, is a thing of the past. Health should not be a barrier in life because it should never stand in the way of goals that you want to achieve. You may find peace of mind after you make changes to your lifestyle.

Improves the environment

A healthy lifestyle does not only benefit you but also everyone around you. As discussed above, regular exercise and eating high-quality food are two ways to help improve the environment by using fewer resources and causing less pollution. If people worldwide live healthier lifestyles, then our planet will be a better place to live in for everyone on it.

A healthy lifestyle provides many benefits while also helping you and everyone else around you to live a happier, more fulfilling life.

Helps you feel better about yourself

Living a healthy lifestyle is one thing you can do to improve your self-esteem. When you eat healthy foods and exercise regularly, you are likely to lose weight and feel more confident in your appearance because of your improved health. You will be proud of having made these positive changes because they will help you feel better about yourself.

While losing weight may appear to be a difficult task, it is not necessary if the proper support system is in place. Changing your diet and exercising regularly can be very easy when other people are also ready to change their lives around them along with yours. You may have more confidence than before and feel better about yourself overall.

EFFECTS OF BAD LIFESTYLE

It is difficult for an individual to avoid the many bad habits of living a fast-paced lifestyle in today's world. People spend every waking hour at work or out with friends and family. When people are busy at work, they eat lunches from vending machines or other places that serve high in fat and sodium. Once people get home from work, many get busy with their children and rarely prepare healthy meals. These factors can contribute to an unhealthy lifestyle, raising the risk of chronic diseases.

Health risks

People who eat high-fat, high-sodium, and sugary foods are often at a higher risk of developing:

Obesity

Due to their hectic lifestyles, people who choose to consume more highly processed foods tend to eat more extra calories, which is the primary cause of obesity.

Heart disease

Overweight people are also at a higher risk of developing heart disease. Obese people, especially those who were metabolically obese, had a higher risk of death. According to a study, metabolically obese means they had above-average blood pressure and cholesterol levels and thus were at an increased risk for heart disease, accounting for 24% of all deaths from cardiovascular diseases.

Diabetes

Individuals who consume a high-sugar, high-fat diet are at an increased risk of developing type 2 diabetes. Individuals who consume a high-sugar, high-fat diet are at an increased risk of developing type 2 diabetes. Studies have shown a diet high in carbohydrates consumed by people who did not have diabetes resulted in higher blood sugar and a greater risk of developing the disease.

While it is unknown which type of diet correlates with a higher risk of diabetes, certain studies have found that LDL cholesterol and triglycerides are correlated with type 2 diabetes.

Cancer

Various types of cancer can be caused by obesity and other bad habits like smoking and drinking alcohol excessively. About 30% of cancers are linked to excess weight, physical inactivity, and poor food choices.

Heart disease is a common risk to overweight, but it is not the only health concern with a bad diet.

Depression

Individuals who consume a lot of sugar and fat have a greater chance of developing depression. Excess consumption of sugars can result in depression by causing the body to become dependent on sugars and make up for the lack of necessary vitamins and minerals.

High cholesterol

High cholesterol is associated with heart disease, but high cholesterol does not always mean that you are at risk for heart disease. A study found that people who had high cholesterol but did not have diseases like high blood pressure or diabetes could still have a higher risk of death due to heart disease.

Gallstones

People who eat foods high in fat and sugar are at a higher risk of developing gallstones, stones formed in the gallbladder. Gallstones can lead to pain and other complications if left untreated.

Poor memory

A high-fat, high-sugar diet can impair the body's ability to break down nutrients, resulting in long-term brain damage. An individual's ability to properly break down nutrients can be impaired by various factors, such as consuming a large amount of fat and sugar or alcohol.

Stroke

People who eat high-fat foods regularly may be more prone to stroke. High blood pressure and cholesterol are two things that contribute to stroke, but a diet high in fat can also increase your chances of having these conditions.

Heartburn

A high-fat, high-sugar diet can cause heartburn, which is a burning sensation in the esophagus caused by stomach acids. Heartburn can be treated with medications in severe cases, but it's also a good idea to try to prevent it in the first place by watching what you eat and drink.

Dementia

An unhealthy diet can cause vascular dementia and Alzheimer's disease, both common causes of dementia. Some research suggests that eating a poor diet can hurt blood vessels in the brain and lead to Alzheimer's disease. People with lower levels of beta-amyloid protein were less likely to develop Alzheimer's disease later in life. People who ate more foods high in fat and protein were less likely to have lower levels of beta-amyloid protein and therefore were more prone to developing Alzheimer's disease.

Acid reflux

Some people experience chronic heartburn and acid reflux due to a diet high in fat and sugar. Acid reflux can cause the esophagus lining to get irritated, making it difficult for food to pass through the digestive system. Eventually, this can lead to loss of appetite, vomiting, nausea, difficulty swallowing, depression, or anxiety.

Infertility

A high-fat, high-sugar diet can increase the risk of infertility, allowing diseases like chlamydia to have an impact on reproductive abilities.

High blood pressure

A study published in the "Hypertension Research" journal showed that people who consumed more than 35 grams of red meat per day were more likely to develop hypertension.

Other risk factors

Overweight individuals have a greater chance of developing any diseases mentioned above, but there are other factors to consider. Another study found that being female and having high blood pressure or high cholesterol doubles your risk of developing Alzheimer's disease. Other risk factors include:

Frequent weight gain

The more often a person gains weight, the greater their risk of developing diabetes and heart disease. People who gain or lose 5-10 pounds on a regular basis have a higher risk of heart disease than those who only gain or lose one pound at a time.

Genetics

Certain genes can increase the chances of having diseases like heart disease. A study showed that having two copies of the gene ApoE4 increased a person's risk of developing heart disease by 50%. Other genes that are believed to increase the risk of heart disease include:

People who have a family member with diabetes or another chronic illness are more likely to develop these diseases themselves in the future. One study published in "Nature Genetics" showed that 51% of people who have one copy of the gene ApoE4 would develop these illnesses compared to only 16% if they do not have a family member with one copy.

Overweight

Obesity is linked to heart disease, diabetes, and high blood pressure. Not only does being overweight increase the risk of having these diseases, but it can cause inflammation in the body that can lead to chronic illness over time.

Overweight pregnant women have a greater chance of developing diabetes during pregnancy and their children when they reach adulthood. Another study found that 10% of children who are obese by age 7 will develop type 2 diabetes compared to 4% of normal-weight children by the same age.

Mild anxiety

Obesity and depression are believed to be linked and may cause both. Mild forms of anxiety can lead to more severe symptoms of depression.

Stress

Hormones are released when the body is stressed, and some research suggests that these hormones may play a role in heart disease and other chronic illnesses. One study published in "Psychosomatic Medicine" found that subjects experiencing stress had higher levels of inflammation, which was a possible cause for heart disease.

Depression

Some studies show that depression can lead to heart disease, but other research suggests that the opposite is true. Depression and stress are linked, but some research suggests that they have different causes. Some research suggests that eating a healthy diet can help reduce symptoms of depression.

When you consider all of these risk factors, it's easy to see why taking preventative measures and understanding how chronic illness develops is so important. To keep from developing heart disease or other illnesses like diabetes, it's essential to understand how your lifestyle affects your health.

Many people experience heartburn, acid reflux, anxiety, and other symptoms that make a living with chronic illness difficult. Treatments for these conditions are available, but diet plays a big role in managing these symptoms.

Each person can make a difference. You can avoid bad habits and create healthy choices, and often, it doesn't take much to make a difference in your life. Look for healthy foods at the grocery store and plan, so you don't have to worry about making quick meals when you get home from work. Stop smoking or drinking alcohol every day, even if your children are not around. Have a plan for exercise that considers how long you will be at work each day or when you have time off in between. Even short walks around the block can help clear your head and give you a sense of accomplishment when you get home tired after a long day of work.

2

THE TOP 10 NATURAL WAYS TO TONE DOWN YOUR BODY

The truth is that there are several quick and simple ways to tone your body the natural way. Although it is correct that losing weight and improving your health requires a significant amount of effort and time, it is all possible with the help of these ten healthy ways to tone down your body.

1. EAT SMALL MEALS

It is possible, however, to tone and slim down without going on a strict diet or engaging in strenuous exercise. It's all about what you eat and how much you eat, which is why a few simple foods can help tone your figure. Eat smaller meals at regular intervals, drink yourself full of water, have healthy snacks ready each morning or evening, and so on. The more you eat, the more calories you will consume.

The recommended size of your meals every day should be about 500 calories. If you are not used to eating so little, you will feel hungry initially, but it will soon go away, given that you eat at least three times a day.

DASH diet: Guide to recommended servings

If you want to lose weight, a diet like the DASH diet can help. The diet stands for Dietary Approaches to Stop Hypertension, which is essentially a heart-healthy eating plan that tells you what food is good for your heart and what foods are bad for you.

It works by maximizing the number of fruits and vegetables you eat, putting a lot of emphasis on whole grains, fish, and seafood, and avoiding sugary foods and excess fats as well as foods high in added sugar.

The DASH diet emphasizes fruits, vegetables, and whole grains. Foods high in saturated fat are restricted, such as fatty meats and full-fat dairy products. In addition, the DASH diet restricts sodium intake to 1,500 to 2,300 milligrams per day.

For two calorie levels of the DASH diet, here are recommended servings from each food group, followed by examples of single-serving sizes for that food group.

Recommended number of servings

Food Group	Daily Servings
Grains (mainly whole grains)	6–8
Meats, poultry, and fish	6 or less
Vegetables	4–5
Low-fat or fat-free milk and milk products	2–3
Fruit	4–5
Nuts, seeds and legumes	3-4 a week
Fats and oils	2–3
	Weekly
Nuts, seeds, dry beans, and peas	4–5
Sweets and added sugars	3 or fewer a week

Source: National Heart, Lung, and Blood Institute

When following the DASH diet, it is critical to eat foods that are:

- Saturated and trans fats are in short supply.
- Potassium, calcium, magnesium, fiber, and protein are all abundant in this dish.
- Sodium is reduced.
- Low fat
- Heart-healthy

2. EXERCISE

Exercising to lose weight is a good way to do so, but exercising helps tone your body as well. You can tone down and trim down by exercising regularly. Finding something you enjoy doing, or at the very least something you believe is feasible, is the key. A good exercise to start with is running, jogging, or brisk walking. It is easy to do, and it helps a lot in toning down your body.

It is critical to exercise. It improves your mood while also strengthening your body. It is the pinnacle of self-care. Don't worry if you're short on time or can't make it to the gym. You can tone and tighten your body by doing a variety of exercises, including these eight.

To create a full-body circuit workout, mix and match these 10 exercises. Begin by performing 10 reps of each exercise for three rounds. Over time, work up to 15 reps for four rounds.

Lunges

Lunges strengthen your legs and gluteus maximus muscles. They'll help you develop sexy legs and buttocks, to put it another way. 0 Lunges also promote functional movement while testing your balance.

Here's how you can do it:

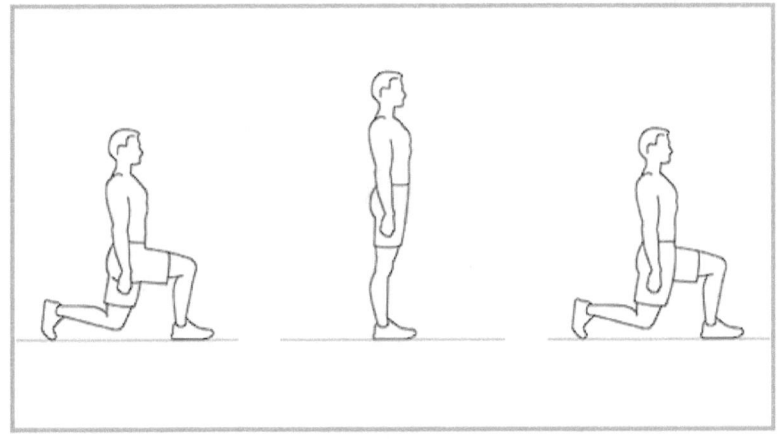

1. Stand tall with your feet together.
2. Lunge forward with your right leg, ensuring that your knees don't go past your toes. If they do, come back to the starting position and move a bit further back next time.
3. When you bring the right foot back to the ground, lunge forward with the left leg. Repeat

15 times on each leg. Save time by holding a hand weight while making lunges more challenging.

Push-Up

The push-up is a must for toning up any area of your body. It's great for building your triceps, shoulders, and chest muscles. Plus, it's one of the best full-body exercises you can do to tone your entire body!

Here's how you can do it:

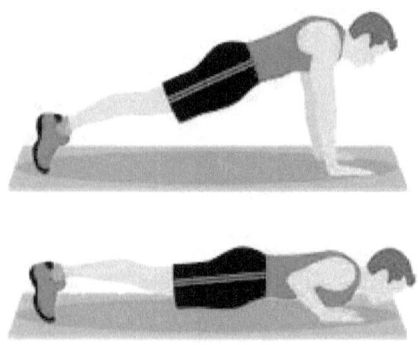

1. Begin on the floor with your hand's shoulder-width apart, and your elbows bent 90 degrees at a 45-degree angle.
2. Keeping your core tight, lower your chest to the floor without letting your back or hips sag.

3. Avoid lowering yourself too fast or pushing upwards until you've reached full extension.
4. Push through the heels and arms to return to the starting position, straightening out completely at the top of each rep.
5. Repeat 15 times on each side for three sets, then take a short break before doing it again.

Leg Lifts

Leg lifts are a relatively easy exercise and great for toning the hip flexor muscles. You can do this exercise from a chair or lying on the floor.

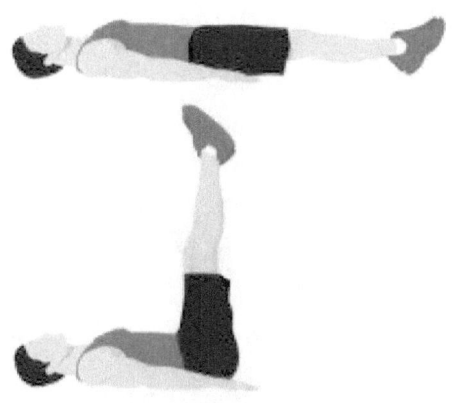

Lift and lower your legs in a circular motion, strengthening your core and gluteus muscles.

Here's how to do it:

1. Press lower back into the floor. While lowering legs, stop once you feel your back lifting off the floor.
2. Lift your legs straight up to the ceiling until your butt is off the floor.
3. Return your legs to a position just above the floor by slowly lowering them. Hold your breath for a moment.
4. Return your legs to their original position. Repeat.

Bicycle Crunches

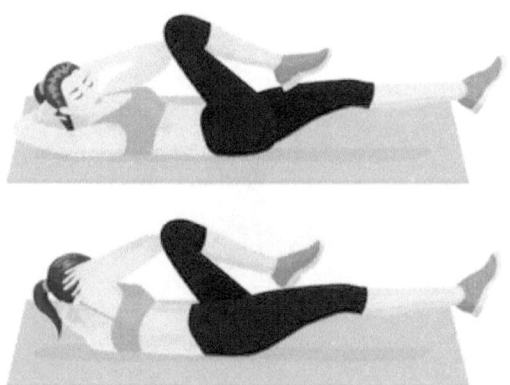

The bicycle crunch is an important exercise to tone the stomach muscles and develop strength and flexibility in those areas.

Here's how you can do it:

1. Placing your hands behind you on the floor. Place your knees close together and extend them straight up towards the ceiling, bending your elbows slightly.
2. Raise and lower your legs in a circular motion to increase tension throughout the muscles targeted during this exercise.
3. Repeat 15 times on each side and then take a short break before doing it again.

Squats

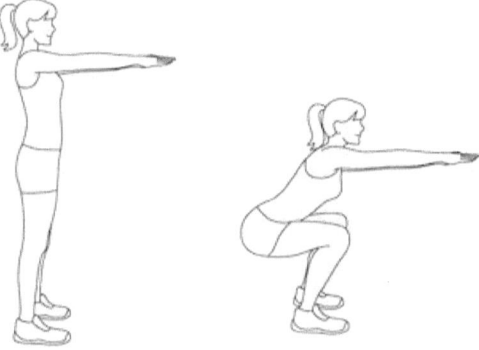

Squats are good for your lower body and core. It also makes your legs and hips more flexible. Squats also help you burn calories because they work out some of your largest muscles.

Here's how you can do it:

1. Stand with your feet shoulder-width apart, keeping your legs straight and core engaged. Your knees should not go beyond your toes. If they do, lower them back to the position in question. For safety reasons, you should always warm up before doing this exercise.
2. Keeping your core tight and shoulders back, begin to lower yourself into a squat position with your thighs parallel to the floor by bending at the waist (think of a runner on their way down).
3. As you lower yourself into your squat, pause briefly, then push back to the starting position.
4. Repeat 15 times on each leg for three sets. You can also perform this exercise as a glute-ham raise, taking it a step further by raising one leg at a time and through the hips to engage the hamstrings fully.

Hip Thrusts

Hip thrusts are effective because they target isolating the glutes and hamstrings often targeted through other exercises. You amp up the intensity and burn more calories by engaging more muscles.

Here's how you can do it:

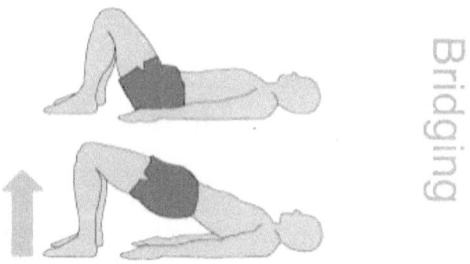

1. Lie on your back, arms overhead, palms facing down, and legs and knees bent to 90 degrees. This is the starting position for your exercise. If you are performing this exercise from a chair or bench, place your feet flat on the floor so that your knees don't go past your toes while performing the movement. Keep an eye on the shoulders while performing these reps to

ensure that they aren't moving too far forward or back during them.

2. Using your glutes, slowly lift your hips off of the floor while keeping your legs as straight as possible. Your torso should be almost perpendicular to the floor and have a slight curve in the low back. The bar should stay directly over the body.
3. As you lift into your hip thrust position, pause at the top of this movement for one second, then lower yourself back down in a slow and controlled manner to complete one rep.
4. Repeat 15 times on each leg for three sets. You can also perform this exercise as a glute-ham raise, taking it a step further by raising one leg at a time and through the hips to engage the hamstrings fully.

Plank

Planks help your body to better compose itself by strengthening a variety of muscle groups as well as the skeletal system.

Here's how you can do it:

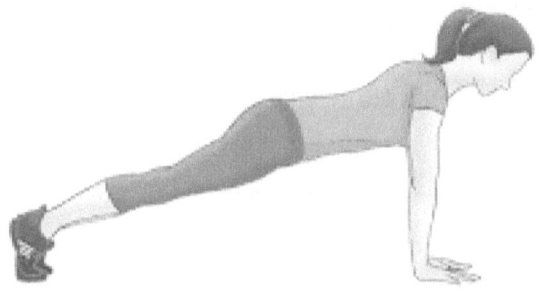

1. Firmly press your palms into the floor and press up from your foundation, widening your shoulder blades as much as possible (this engages your upper back). Consider lifting your back of your neck toward the ceiling while keeping your neck lengthened forward (i.e., don't look down). Allowing your shoulders to scrunch or shrug up toward your ears is not a good idea.
2. Your arms should feel tense but not strained—not as if they're about to snap.

3. A plank will work your abs, but your legs should also feel the burn. If they don't, they'll push through your heels and into the floor with the balls of your feet. Engage your quadriceps (also known as thighs) and squeeze your glutes (butt muscles) together to activate the muscles in your lower body. Consider the muscles in your buttocks tightly wrapping around your sit bones.
4. While we're on the subject of gluteals, keep your booty low during a plank—not lifted toward the sky. A straight line, rather than a triangle, should appeal to your body.
5. Don't forget to take a deep breath. Your lungs should not stop moving just because you're challenging your muscles to maintain contraction. Remember to inhale and exhale in a rhythmic pattern throughout your plank. In fact, if you're not one to watch the clock—but are one to forget to breathe—timing your plank by breaths in and out might be a good idea. If you're just getting started, try holding a plank for five breaths in and out before releasing.

Sit-ups

Sit-ups are a classic exercise that targets the abdominal muscles, developing strength and flexibility in that region of the body.

Here's how you can do it:

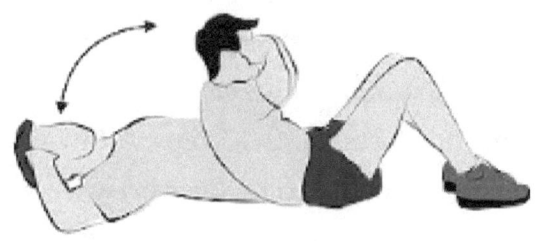

© CanStockPhoto.com

1. Begin by bending your knees and lying on your back. Sit-ups are most effective when performed on a soft surface, such as a mattress. Maintain a 90-degree angle with your knees bent and your feet flat on the floor.
2. Place your fingertips behind your ears. You should have your elbows bent and pointing out to the sides. When doing sit-ups, cupping the back of your ears with your fingertips rather than placing them on the back of your head can

help you avoid pulling yourself up by your neck.
3. Raise your torso as close as possible to your thighs. Keep your feet flat on the floor and move in a smooth, steady motion. Once you've completed lifting your torso, your lower back should be elevated off the floor.
4. Lower your torso to the floor to return to the starting position. Lower your torso in a smooth and steady motion, just as you did when you lifted it up to your thighs.
5. Perform three sets of 10-15 reps. Allow your body about a minute to recover between sets. If you're having trouble maintaining proper form, reduce the number of sit-ups you do until you're stronger.

3. DRINK MORE WATER

Increased water consumption can boost metabolism, reduce inflammation, and jump-start digestion.

Reasons why drinking more water may aid in weight loss include the following:

1. Water can help you lose weight by suppressing your appetite naturally

When you realize you're hungry, your first instinct may be to go out and get something to eat. However, eating may not be the solution. "The brain often confuses thirst, which is triggered by mild dehydration, with hunger," says Melina Jampolis, an internist and board-certified physician nutrition specialist. "If you are low in water rather than calories, you may be able to reduce your appetite by drinking water."

Additionally, water can help you feel fuller faster by stretching your stomach as it quickly passes through your system. "This sends fullness signals to your brain," Jampolis explains.

Consuming water shortly before eating may help decrease food intake. According to a small 2016 study, people who drank two glasses of water immediately before a meal consumed 22% less food than those who did not.

Two cups should be enough to fill your stomach to the point where your brain registers fullness.

2. Water can increase your metabolism, which burns calories

According to the National Academy of Sciences, the amount of water you drink each day directly correlates with how many calories you burn. The more fluids your body takes in, the more likely you are to increase your metabolism and begin burning calories, even when you're at rest.

Drinking enough water may also reduce inflammation to keep you feeling energetic and help you lose weight.

3. Water can kick-start digestion and prevent overeating

Drinking water first thing in the morning assists your body in eliminating any excess toxins that may have accumulated in the stomach while you slept. When you wake up, your body has to work to digest food and fight off any diseases and infections it may have come into contact with while asleep.

This makes water a good option for helping fight everything from heart disease to cancer to inflammation. Drinking water increased the activity of hydroxyl radical enzymes in subjects by 37%. This is important because these enzymes are often linked with aging and various diseases, including heart disease and arthritis.

4. Water can reduce inflammation, boost brain function, and make muscles more efficient

Inflammation is at the root of a slew of health issues. For example, chronic inflammation can lead to heart disease and diabetes. Drinking water can help people with joint pain and other inflammatory conditions.

Water can also help keep your brain sharp by improving overall brain function and forming memories. For example, when researchers supplemented older adults' diets with water for 2 weeks, they found that their memory improved by 25 percent, and their reaction time was faster.

5. During exercise, it is beneficial to drink water

Drinking water before and during exercise can aid performance by replacing the fluids your body loses due to sweat, maintaining electrolyte balance, and avoiding dehydration.

Drinking water during exercise can also help you lose weight. One study found that runners lost an average of 5 pounds per year by drinking just 25 ounces of water before and during each workout, which was enough to substitute the calories they burned from running.

6. Water aids in the removal of waste from the body

Your body automatically flushes waste out of its system as you go about your day. However, some waste can stay in the body for long periods, leading to health issues like heart disease and cancer. Consuming water aids in the elimination of toxins from the body by causing them to pass through your urine.

Water also aids in flushing fluids from your lungs, which can be important for removing more powerful toxins, such as heavy metals and certain chemicals.

7. Water can help prevent dehydration by keeping you feeling full and well-hydrated

Dehydration is just like thirst in that it's often confused with hunger - water helps fill you up but doesn't necessarily keep you full. This can lead many to overeat, which can lead to weight gain.

Drinking enough water throughout the day will help you stay hydrated and feel full.

Water makes up 70% of your total body weight and is the most abundant substance in your body. More than 60% of your brain is made up of water, and more than 90% of your digestive tract is made up of water. Water is required for your body to function properly, as it is used to take in nutrients, remove waste products, regulate blood pressure and temperature, and transport nutrients to cells.

If you suffer from excess weight, you should consume 1-2 liters of water every day (preferably 1.5 liters).

Weight loss can be found in many different forms, but the one thing that keeps most people away from it is time for exercise, planning meals, and just the sheer amount of work needed to keep on top of everything.

Losing weight doesn't have to cost a fortune or come with crazy stipulations.

4. CONSUME FOODS HIGH IN FIBER.

You will see many benefits from eating fiber, but one of the biggest is increased weight loss. You might not lose weight immediately, but your body will eventually adjust to having more fiber in your diet, which will help reduce cravings. Over time, you'll notice that your body feels less hungry, and you eat less overall, which reduces cravings.

The simplest way to eat more fiber is to increase the amount of fruit and vegetables you eat. By doing so, you will be eating even more fiber.

Dietary fiber is an important part of maintaining a healthy lifestyle. Plants, fruits, vegetables, legumes, and whole-grain parts that your body can't fully digest are examples of dietary fiber, also known as roughage. Dietary fiber passes largely undigested through your digestive tract until it reaches the colon or large intestine, where microbiota ferments some fibers.

By regulating bowel movements, softening stool, and reducing constipation, a high-fiber diet can help maintain bowel health. High-fiber foods are also more filling than low-fiber foods, so they can help you feel satisfied.

Different types of fiber foods

Soluble

Dietary fiber that dissolves in water and absorbs water during digestion to form a gel-like substance is known as soluble dietary fiber. Oats, peas, beans, fruits, and barley are high in soluble fiber.

Insoluble

Dietary fiber that does not dissolve in water and is not broken down by enzymes during absorption is known as insoluble dietary fiber. Insoluble fiber is, for example, the cellulose that makes up fruit and vegetable cell walls (though other plant components like lignin or waxes are also insoluble). Some examples of high insoluble fiber foods are whole-grain bread and cereals, wheat bran, nuts (particularly peanuts), popcorn, and brown rice.

Incorporate high-fiber foods into your daily routine, including regular meals, snacks, and smoothies. It's also important to start slowly and gradually increasing your dietary fiber intake rather than all at once if you're trying to increase fiber in your diet. The most important thing is not stopping eating fiber but lightly increasing your intake.

The following foods are high in fiber and can be included in your diet:

Beans

In soups, stews, and salads, lentils and other beans are an easy way to get fiber into your diet. Some beans, such as edamame (a steamed soybean), can even be used as a fiber-rich snack. A half-cup serving of shelled edamame contains 9 grams of fiber. Is there a bonus? All of these are also good sources of plant protein. Some bakers have even started using beans or bean flours in their baked goods, proving that quality cakes can still be made with beans.

Oatmeal

Oatmeal is a wonderful way to start your day. It's quick and easy to make, but remember that it has small amounts of calories and most people eat more than its actual serving size leads you to believe. A half-cup serving of oatmeal has 3 grams of fiber.

Potatoes

Potatoes are an excellent addition to a healthy diet plan because they are one of the world's primary carbohydrate sources. They can be eaten in side dishes like mashed potatoes, boiled, or baked. You can also eat them as a snack by themselves, just not French fries. The fiber content of a medium-baked potato with the skin on is 10 grams.

Whole grains

Whole-grain bread and tortillas are some of the best whole-grain sources out there. Unfortunately, processed foods tend to be made from refined grains that don't contain their full set of nutrients, so it's a good idea to limit your consumption of these types of foods and choose whole grains instead. Whole grains are healthier than other forms of bread and tortillas, so you should always choose these over refined ones. Overly milled whole grains can be difficult to chew, so go for the type that has been milled a bit coarser. If you want to make sure you're getting your daily fiber, look at the next two sources on this list.

Vegetables

When you eat your vegetables, you get your fiber. Vegetables also provide a wide range of vitamins and minerals that keep you healthy. If you can, eat a variety of vegetables so that you're getting the most vitamins, minerals, and fiber possible. One cup of leafy greens like kale contains 2 grams of fiber.

Fruit

Fresh fruit provides an already natural source of vitamins and minerals and health-benefiting dietary fiber. According to studies, individuals who consumed three or more servings per day were 24 percent less likely to develop constipation than those who consumed one or fewer servings per day. A half-cup serving of apple slices contains 1.6 grams of fiber.

Nuts

Nuts, also known as seeds, are a great source of healthy fats, vitamins, and minerals but are also a wonderful way to get your daily intake of dietary fiber in your diet. They provide a very nice snack when eaten with an apple or banana for the perfect afternoon pick-me-up. A half-cup serving of chopped nuts has 4 grams of fiber.

Dried fruits

Dried fruits are treated with heat to preserve their mineral content and flavor for eating as a snack or dessert after crushing them up into smaller pieces like raisins or apricots (about ½ cup) are a great source of fiber. An apple or orange slice (1 slice of fruit) provides 1 gram of fiber.

Dietary fibers are very important in maintaining a healthy lifestyle by maintaining bowel function and reducing constipation while providing your body with important nutrients and vitamins. Dietary fibers can also be added to many different types of foods during cooking to give them a richer flavor and make them healthier.

5. WATCH YOUR DAILY INTAKE OF SALT

Salt is a great taste enhancer, but too much can wreak havoc on your body. Excess salt consumption can result in hypertension, obesity, osteoporosis, and kidney disease. High blood pressure, obesity, osteoporosis, and kidney disease can all be caused by too much salt. And it's not as if you even need the extra salt: Most people are getting more than enough through processed foods, restaurant meals, and fast foods.

You can reduce your salt intake by doing the following:

- Use fresh meats instead of pre-packaged meats. Natural sodium is present in fresh cuts of beef, chicken, and pork, but it is far less than the extra sodium added during processing in bacon and ham. If a food item lasts for days or weeks in the fridge, it's a sign that the sodium content is too high.
- Instead of table salt, use sea salt or kosher salt. Most of our sodium comes from the processed foods we eat, and it's in the form of sodium chloride. If you can't find sea or kosher salt at the supermarket, grab some Himalayan salt and grind it up with a coffee grinder to get a coarse kind that will add more flavor but will not be as high in sodium as table salt.
- Cut down on your use of condiments and spreads like ketchup, soy sauce, barbecue sauce, and salad dressing that are high in sodium, such as balsamic vinegar. You can also use homemade condiments such as hummus instead of ketchup or barbecue sauce.

- Avoid processed meats like bacon, hot dogs, salami, and lunch meats. If you must have a slice or two, opt for turkey bacon or turkey ham instead of the standard variety.
- Cut down on the amount of bread and potatoes you eat. Nobody eats just one small slice of bread, and a large baked potato can have thousands of milligrams of sodium in it.
- Choose unsalted nuts or seeds over salted ones. While eating a handful of nuts here and there will not make much of a difference, if you are eating them as snacks throughout the day or if you are using them in recipes or meals as an ingredient, opt for the unsalted variety instead of their saltier counterparts.
- Use fresh herbs like parsley and mint to add flavor to your dishes instead of salt while cooking them and before serving them.
- Limit your consumption of processed foods and fast foods as much as possible.
- Choose low-sodium soups and broths instead of high-sodium varieties such as canned broth and bouillon cubes. Homemade soups are a great way to test out all the flavors you want while keeping sodium in check.
- When cooking rice, potatoes, bread, or quinoa,

substitute lemon juice or apple cider vinegar for salt to enhance the flavor without adding additional sodium.
- Make your own stocks. Homemade stock is a great way to add extra flavor to your recipes, and it can be made with low-sodium chicken, beef, pork, lamb, or vegetable stock.
- When cooking, flavor your meals with herbs and spices rather than salt. Spices like bay leaves, cloves, coriander seeds, cinnamon sticks, cumin seeds, fennel seeds, garlic powder, and onion powder are great ways to add flavor without adding sodium.
- Eat more fresh fruits and vegetables for added flavor.
- Consume water rather than sugary beverages such as soda or fruit juice, as these beverages contain salt that you would otherwise get from a bag of chips.

Salts can be found in many different foods, and they are used to flavor them to make them taste better. If you think that salt is just a seasoning, you may want to reconsider because your body isn't really getting the full benefit of these minerals since they get "hidden" in your food. Once you start eating a healthier diet, your body will start working with what it is being offered, which means that you will be getting less salt in it.

6. HAVE A CRUNCHY SNACK DAILY TO SATISFY YOUR NEED FOR SOMETHING CREAKY

Crunchy snacks like nuts and seeds are full of nutrients, but some people may have difficulty eating them because they aren't always the easiest to chew. Instead of avoiding them, chew on them for longer than normal to help get greater benefits from the nutrients. If you still find that difficult, add more of these foods into your diet in other ways. You can bake with nuts and seeds and use them in your breakfast cereal, or add raw vegetables like radishes, cucumbers, or carrots with some sprouts and pair it with hummus or dip made from tahini or other nut and oil-based spreads.

If you're worried about eating too much extra fat or calories from nuts, seeds, and nut butter, do not be. People who eat a lot of nuts have a lower risk of heart disease and type 2 diabetes and can lose more weight.

7. CONSUME LESS RED MEAT AND DAIRY PRODUCTS

These foods may have a high amount of lipids and saturated fats, which can contribute to an increase in bad cholesterol levels. Beans, chickpeas, and lentils can be used in place of greens if you're concerned about protein. The Soyfoods Association says that vegans need 60 to 80 grams of protein per day at the minimum, or 1 gram per kilogram of bodyweight if you want to get into the profound details of how much protein you need per day.

Many people who eat a vegan diet also tend to have higher levels of good cholesterol, which helps them avoid developing heart disease. There are many different ways to get adequate protein. The list includes tofu, tempeh, soy milk, soy yogurt, plant-based meats (e.g., seitan or tofu), pulses (e.g., chickpeas or lentils), nut butter made from pulses like cashew and pumpkin seeds (e.g., sunflower and sesame seeds, pumpkin seeds, almonds, walnuts, peanuts), fortified cereals, legumes (lentils, chickpeas or beans) and green veggies.

8. EAT MORE WHOLE GRAINS

Whole grains contain a lot of B vitamins, which help to protect cells and maintain a healthy metabolism. Whole grains include things like wheat berries and amaranth. However, be careful about picking up the wrong products labeled as whole grain but really aren't because they can contain more sugar than you probably care to have in your diet.

You may not yet understand the distinction between whole-grain and refined grain foods, but chances are you're already eating some whole-grain foods. You're eating whole-grain foods if you have a bowl of oatmeal for breakfast or popcorn at the movies. The first thing to know about whole grains is that they contain more nutrients than refined grains, are healthier for your heart, and aid in weight loss.

The entire grain seed is used to make whole-grain foods. When a whole grain, such as wheat or rice, is crushed, cracked, or cooked in the processing process, parts of the grain kernel, such as the bran and germ, are lost, along with some fiber, vitamins, and minerals. However, you can find whole-grain products that aren't just wheat or rice with some careful shopping.

The Advantages of Whole Grain Foods

Whole grains should be included in your diet if you are trying to lose weight or eat a heart-healthy diet. One of the best examples of choosing quality calories over empty calories is whole grains.

Weight loss

Whole grains reduce the risk of obesity and cholesterol.

Health benefits

Studies on whole grains have shown that they can reduce the risk of several chronic diseases, such as diabetes and heart disease. They are also shown to increase satiety and metabolism.

Nutritional benefits

Whole grains have high amounts of fiber, which can help you feel full and satisfied. Whole grains also contain healthy fats and a high amount of protein compared to refined grains. There are many other nutritional benefits to eating whole grains, including vitamins B and E, folate (folic acid), iron, zinc, magnesium, potassium, and selenium.

9. BE REALISTIC

Losing weight is exhausting and not always easy. There will be days where you feel like you have no energy, but you have to push through it. If you're on a raw vegetable diet, your body may begin to shut down due to a lack of energy to deal with what's being thrown at it. It's critical to avoid feeling guilty about your emotions and instead concentrate on the fact that you're working to better yourself and your body.

10. GET ENOUGH SLEEP

It's challenging to lose weight and even more challenging to keep it off. Numerous potential links have emerged highlighting the potential weight loss benefits of getting a good night's sleep and the negative health consequences of sleep deprivation, despite the medical community's ongoing efforts to decipher the complicated relationship between sleep and body weight.

Sleep and Weight: Is There a Link?

While the exact nature of this relationship is still being debated in the medical community, existing research indicates a positive link between good sleep and healthy body weight.

There's still a lot to learn about the complicated relationship between sleep and weight. Several hypotheses provide avenues for further investigation in the hopes of improving our understanding of the relationship between weight and sleep, which will lead to less obesity and more effective weight-loss methods.

One popular theory about the link between weight and sleep is that sleep influences appetite. Appetite is controlled by neurotransmitters, which are chemical messengers that allow neurons (nerve cells) to communicate.

Ghrelin and leptin are neurotransmitters thought to play a role in appetite. Ghrelin promotes hunger, while leptin aids in feeling satisfied. The body naturally regulates the levels of these neurotransmitters throughout the day, signaling the need for calories.

In addition to appetite-controlling neurotransmitters, people are also thought to naturally vary their caloric intake over the course of the day. Greater weight gain is associated with reduced sleep duration, which may increase ghrelin levels, leading to increased appetite and reduced satiety.

A part of the brain regulates ghrelin and leptin levels. In one study, subjects were allowed 2 hours less sleep per night for 6 days in a row. A significant reduction was found in leptin levels, while ghrelin levels (appetite-regulating) increased significantly after only 2 nights of restricted sleep.

Another common theory about the link between weight and sleep is that a lack of sleep may compromise the brain's ability to use insulin properly. Insulin is a hormone that promotes glucose or blood sugar uptake by cells.

Too little insulin results in high blood sugar and can lead to diabetes, which increases the risk for obesity, cardiovascular disease, hypertension (high blood pressure), and more. Because of the relationship between high blood sugar and weight gain, some researchers believe a lack of proper insulin regulation may be an underlying cause of weight gain in people who get too little sleep.

Taken together, these and other research findings suggest a potential link between poor sleep patterns and weight gain. The true nature of this relationship, however, is still unclear.

While it may seem like a daunting task to lose weight and get enough sleep simultaneously, it's not impossible. Losing weight is like any other habit: You must be passionate about making changes for yourself. Since most overweight people are not necessarily aware that they have a problem, it takes effort and fast results to get your mind and body on board with healthier habits. Stay positive if you have tried other diets only to gain more weight. Try this diet — if you stick with it, you will likely see results in as little as a week.

Above all else, remember to choose your foods wisely and quit overindulging in sugary, fatty, salty, and processed foods. Simultaneously, it is critical to maintain healthy body weight and muscle mass through a variety of high-quality proteins, complex carbohydrates, healthy fats (nuts and olive oil), fruits, and vegetables.

Always seek medical advice before beginning any diet or exercise program.

3

HEALTH BENEFITS OF A BALANCED DIET

It's no coincidence that the rapid rise in obesity coincided with the increased availability of highly processed foods.

Although convenient, highly processed foods are high in calories, low in nutrients, and increase your risk of various diseases.

On the contrary, natural foods are packed with nutrients and fewer calories.

By choosing to eat a balanced diet, you will be able to:

1. Beat Obesity Naturally

You're going to lose weight when you cut certain types of junk food from your diet. However, what's not as obvious is that natural foods are also good for you, like fruits and vegetables. They contain essential vitamins, minerals, antioxidants, and fiber to promote weight loss. To put it simply: a balanced diet keeps the body functioning optimally while toning down unwanted pounds.

2. Get Essential Nutrients

Essential nutrients are those that your body requires for normal functioning but cannot produce independently. The body may lack essential nutrients if you don't eat enough fruits and vegetables rich in these materials. A deficiency in essential nutrients can cause serious health problems like headaches, anxiety, fatigue, and muscle pain. A healthy diet helps prevent this from happening.

3. Boost Your Immune System

The essential vitamins and minerals found in natural foods help develop a strong immune system so you can fend off infections and illnesses. A balanced diet keeps your immune system at its peak so it can protect you from disease-causing microorganisms like bacteria, viruses, and parasites.

4. Decrease Your Risk of Cancer

Anticancer agents and antioxidants are abundant in foods that have undergone little to no processing, helping to protect cells from environmental damage. This helps lower your risk of developing cancer cells, especially if you eat them daily. A balanced diet ensures your body gets enough healthy foods to lower your chances of developing cancer.

5. Maintain Bone Health

Osteoporosis, which weakens and fractures the bones of postmenopausal women, is one of the most serious consequences of an unhealthy diet. The right balance of vitamins and minerals found in natural foods promotes bone strength and health so that you can avoid fractures in old age.

6. Avoid Diabetes

Excess weight and poor diet can cause insulin resistance, which can lead to type 2 diabetes, characterized by high blood glucose levels that damage body organs. A balanced diet helps you avoid type 2 diabetes by assisting you in losing excess weight, which enables your body to regulate blood glucose levels.

7. Keep Your Heart Healthy

A balanced diet drastically lowers your risk of developing cardiovascular diseases, including heart disease and stroke. A healthy diet also keeps your cholesterol levels at desirable levels to lower your heart attack and stroke risk.

8. Lower Your Cholesterol Levels

Feeling exhausted, anxious, and having mood swings are not good signs if they stem from high cholesterol levels. A balanced diet keeps your cholesterol levels under control to decrease your risk of developing cardiovascular diseases.

9. Reduce Inflammation

One of the major causes of inflammation is stress, which leads to an unhealthy diet. A balanced diet helps reduce inflammation by providing you with essential nutrients that can prevent this condition from arising in the first place.

HOW MUCH PROTEIN, FAT, AND CARBOHYDRATES SHOULD I HAVE?

There are macronutrients and micronutrients when it comes to nutrition. Fats, carbohydrates, and protein are the "big three" macronutrients (macros). When consumed in the right proportions, these three macronutrients can help you lose weight, improve your health, and feel better overall.

MACRONUTRIENT	Recommended Ranges
Carbohydrate	45-65%
Protein	10-35%
Fats	20-35%

Most adults should aim for a 45-65 percent carbohydrate, 10-35 percent protein, and 20-35 percent fat ratio in their diets. (If you're trying to lose weight, adjust the percentages to 10-30% carbohydrates, 40-50% protein, and 30-40% fat.)

Traditional calorie counting has several flaws, one of which is that it ignores the quality of the food you consume. While portion control alone may work in the short term, your self-control will eventually break down unless you're eating nutrient-dense foods that leave you satisfied. More information on how to get the most out of the macronutrients each day can be found below:

Carbohydrates

Although carbs have recently become the subject of some controversy, they are still a crucial component of our diets. To maintain optimal health and weight, the American Heart Association recommends that most adults consume 45-65 percent carbohydrates each day.

One serving of a simple carbohydrate has four calories (compared to 3 for fat and 1 for protein). Carbohydrates supply us with energy and important nutrients such as fiber, vitamins, minerals, and antioxidants. They also help us feel fuller, thus helping us eat less throughout the day.

The body converts carbohydrates to glucose, a monosaccharide that cells use for energy. Simple carbs are processed quickly by the body to produce energy; therefore, they can cause spikes and dips in your blood sugars. But on the other side, complex carbs, such as those found in whole-grain bread, brown rice, legumes, whole fruits, and vegetables, are digested much more slowly and contain fewer calories in total than simple carbs. Complex carbs provide long-lasting fuel to keep you going all day long while maintaining steady blood sugar levels (which can help prevent overeating) and higher metabolism.

Another way to determine if carbohydrates are right for you is to eat a high-carb meal and measure your blood sugar and insulin levels after. If you don't feel like having something, try the high-carb meal again in the next couple of hours, as your body may not be done processing it yet. This is especially useful if you're on a low-carb diet.

Unprocessed or minimally processed starches like potatoes or yams, vegetables, fruits, and beans are the healthiest sources of carbohydrates. They help you stay healthy by providing vitamins, minerals, fiber, and various other nutrients. Bread, pasta, pastries, sodas, and other processed or refined foods are all unhealthy sources of carbohydrates. These foods contain high-glycemic-index carbohydrates that contribute to weight gain, hormone imbalance, diabetes, and heart disease. Your goal should be to consume carbohydrates from whole foods such as vegetables, legumes, and fruit, that are minimally processed, so they contain more vitamins, minerals, and nutrients.

Fats

The body needs fats to function properly, making them an important part of a balanced diet. Fats also contribute to good health because they help build cells and deliver essential nutrients such as Vitamin D and cholesterol. Essential fats (omega-3's) are found in fatty fish, nuts and seeds, olive oil, avocados, flaxseeds, and coconuts. Omega-6 oils can be found in animal sources such as chicken or fish products or vegetable oils like corn oil.

Fats are made of triglycerides, which contain three fatty acids attached to a molecule to glycerol. The fatty acids contained in the fats vary in terms of length saturation and are linked together.

The number of double bonds in a fat molecule's molecular structure indicates whether it is saturated or unsaturated. At room temperature, saturated fats are solid. When consumed instead of saturated fats, unsaturated fats are usually liquid at room temperature and are considered healthier than saturated fats because they lower overall cholesterol levels.

Fat is one of the three macronutrients needed for good health, along with carbohydrates and proteins. The ideal amount of fat in a diet is essential to maintain good health.

Don't be afraid of fats. Fats help you feel full, keep your energy up, and boost the absorption of some vitamins. Good fats are necessary for your body's functions and must be consumed regularly to prevent deficiencies. Unfortunately, processed foods often contain trans-fat (partially hydrogenated fats), created when liquid oils are changed into trans-fats through hydrogenation. Trans-fat increases cardiovascular disease, obesity, diabetes, and osteoporosis. Eat these foods sparingly as part of a healthy diet.

Protein

Protein is needed to build, repair, and maintain body tissue. That's why we get protein from eating meat, fish, poultry, tofu, and other plant foods. Protein also increases metabolism to help burn fat for fuel or muscle for physical activity. The recommended daily amount of protein is about 50-60 grams per day for women and men between the ages of 19 and 50; slightly more than 100 grams per day for men over age 50.

Most Americans eat enough protein in their diets, so you probably don't need to worry about eating more of it. However, if your body cannot absorb enough protein or if you're an athlete that needs extra protein, supplements or foods with additional protein may be necessary.

Athletes and bodybuilders often need to increase their daily protein intake for muscle building and repair. Protein powders and shakes are convenient for people who don't have time to prepare food or that want an alternative to eating meat all the time. To gain lean muscle mass, a dieter must consume plenty of calories so that excess protein is used for building lean tissue rather than stored as fat.

Learning to prepare healthy meals that incorporate protein can be a challenge. Protein helps us build and maintain muscle, but it also turns into glucose in the bloodstream, raising insulin levels and inhibiting fat burning. Eat your protein with good fats like nuts or avocado to help keep your insulin levels down and increase energy expenditure.

Many women's diets are deficient in protein, resulting in osteoporosis as a result of the body's inability to absorb enough calcium from food.

By consuming lean meats, fish, eggs, whole milk, dairy products, and certain plant foods such as dried beans and peas, you can make sure that you meet your daily protein needs without consuming excess calories from animal sources of fat.

MICRONUTRIENTS

Micronutrients are substances that the body requires in small amounts in order to carry out normal physiological functions. Micronutrients include minerals and vitamins, vital to keeping your body functioning properly.

Vitamins, minerals, and phytochemicals are essential for health because they help your body maintain normal functions, especially metabolism. Other nutrients are necessary for proper function but not necessary. Nutrients come from natural foods (vegetables, fruits, nuts, seeds, grass-fed meats) and processed foods (cereals). RDAs (Recommended Dietary Allowances) are daily micronutrients determined by scientists at the Institute of Medicine based on age, gender, and life stage. It's important to remember that these recommended values are meant to prevent deficiencies and the diseases and conditions that go along with them, not necessarily to promote longevity and optimal health.

Benchmarks of a well-balanced diet include:

Vitamins or Minerals	Recommended Dietary Allowance (RDA) for Men	Recommended Dietary Allowance (RDA) for Women
Fiber	38g	25g
Vitamin C	90mg	75mg
Calcium	1000mg	1200mg
Iron	18mg	18mg
Magnesium	420mg	380mg
Zinc	11mg	8mg
Sodium	1500mg	1000mg
Chloride	2300mg	2000mg

Potassium	4700mg	3500mg
Sulfur	1.5mg	1mg
Phosphorus	700 mg	700 mg

Fiber

A vital component of a well-balanced diet. Fiber is not digested or absorbed, but it helps to regulate bowel movements and blood sugar levels, which helps in the prevention of diabetes and heart disease. Fiber also promotes good digestive health by helping you feel satisfied after eating and metabolize food more efficiently than when not eating enough fiber. Whole fruits, vegetables, legumes, and grains are high in fiber.

Vitamin C

It helps with healthy tissue growth and repair; immune function helps fight off infections promotes healthy skin and hair. This compound is found in oranges and lemons, as well as spinach and broccoli.

Calcium

It helps build bones and teeth, as well as nerve function. According to some studies, people who consume more dairy have fewer bone breaks as a result of falls or fractures than those who consume less dairy. Found in dairy products, dark green vegetables such as spinach or kale, and sardines.

Iron

Helps carry oxygen to the cells. Iron deficiency causes anemia. Found in organ meats, leafy greens, fiber-rich foods like whole grains and beans, fortified cereals, dried apricots, and raisins.

Magnesium

Aids in bone development and maintenance; muscle function; keeps nerves functioning properly; helps with the proper development of teeth, hair, and nails. Found in leafy greens, green veggies like broccoli and spinach, nuts such as almonds or cashews.

Zinc

Promotes strong immune function; helps wounds heal; builds proteins for cell division; a component of DNA and RNA in cells, and wound healing. Found in meats, whole grains, nuts and seeds, and grain-based desserts.

Sodium

It is important for nerve impulse transmission throughout the body. It also helps regulate heart rhythm, helps the body maintain fluid balance, a component of sweat, saliva, tears, and stomach fluid;

helps the body maintain blood pressure. Found in table salt (sodium chloride) or high-sodium foods such as canned goods (high-sodium foods expand when heated) or fast foods.

Chloride

An essential component of hydrochloric acid (HCl) in the stomach; regulates pH. Found in table salt (sodium chloride) or high-sodium foods such as canned goods (high-sodium foods expand when heated) or fast foods.

Potassium

It helps regulate body fluids, including blood pressure and body temperature; helps nerve and muscle function; regulates heartbeat; keeps water and nutrients in cells, including sodium. Found in fresh fruits such as bananas, oranges, cantaloupe, and vegetables such as tomatoes, mushrooms, and spinach.

Sulfur (or sulfur, sulfate, sulfide, or bisulfite)

An important component of many enzymes; helps keep bones strong; prevents tooth decay. Found in meat, eggs, legumes, and whole grains.

Phosphorus

It is involved in bone formation; helps regulate blood glucose levels; helps maintain the body's acid-base balance by playing a role in maintaining the level of bicarbonate ions in the bloodstream that keeps normal pH levels; helps with muscle and nerve function, including the brain. Found in meat, fish, eggs, legumes, nuts, seeds, and whole grains.

A well-balanced diet is crucial to maintaining a healthy lifestyle. It is important to know that many factors, including age, gender, medical conditions, and their environment, can change the necessity of nutrients needed to keep the body fit. Sometimes people eat well but are still not getting the necessary amounts of food that their body needs. This can be due to too little time to prepare healthy meals or a lack of money for healthy groceries. Often poor eating habits are caused by social norms such as eating fast food on the run or skipping meals in order to save money. Balancing your diet is crucial to maintaining good health and living longer.

4

WEEKLY MENU PLAN FOR WEIGHT LOSS

Many weight loss meal plans are available online, and deciding which one to follow can be difficult. It does not require calorie counting and other tricky calculations. A diet rich in whole foods can help you feel full longer, and this should translate into fewer snacking episodes and less over-eating at meals. The diet plan outlined here is based on the principles of healthy eating, which includes fresh vegetables, fruits, whole grains, lean meat, poultry, seafood, and beans.

HOW TO MAKE A WEIGHT-LOSS MEAL PLAN

Meals should be planned around a person's specific requirements. They should think about:

- How much weight they need to lose
- How active they are
- Any health-related dietary restrictions
- Any personal, cultural, or religious dietary restrictions
- How much time do they have available for food preparation and shopping
- The difficulty of the recipes and their level of cooking expertise
- Whether the meal plan should include other family members

This menu plan is based on a daily calorie requirement appropriate for weight loss. The number of calories needed varies with each individual, as do the nutrients and other ingredients in a healthy meal plan.

The sample menu drawn up here contains a 1,600 calorie allowance per day, which is appropriate for most moderately active adults who need to lose weight. This activity level allows for some leeway in the types of food and beverages consumed and the number of servings per day while still allowing weight loss to occur. To achieve more substantial weight loss requires a lower caloric intake than 1,600 calories (or even 1,200 calories) per day, along with an exercise program that burns several hundred calories per day.

BREAKFAST RECIPES

Scrambled egg with spinach & tomato (Day 1)

Ingredients

- 1 large egg
- 3 tablespoons of low-fat milk
- 2 tablespoons of diced red onion
- 1/4 teaspoon salt
- 1/4 teaspoon black pepper
- 2 tablespoons of chopped fresh cilantro
- 5 ounces of spinach leaves
- 1 medium (approximately 6 ounces) tomato, cut into wedges. (optional)

Directions

1. Beat the egg with the milk until blended.
2. Add salt, pepper, and onion, then stir in the spinach and cilantro.
3. Drizzle olive oil into a nonstick skillet over medium heat.

4. Pour in the egg mixture and cook until lightly brown on one side, then flip and continue to cook until thoroughly cooked through.
5. Top with tomato wedges if desired.

Oatmeal with brown sugar and milk (Day 2)

Ingredients

- 1/4 cup steel-cut oats
- 3/4 cup of fat-free milk
- 1 small banana, sliced
- 2 tsp brown sugar, or more to taste
- 5 small almonds, chopped. (optional)

Directions

1. Bring 1 cup of water and the oats to a boil in a saucepan.
2. Reduce to low heat, cover, and cook for 5 minutes, or until oats are tender.
3. Turn off the heat and set it aside for 5 minutes.
4. Stir in the milk until combined.
5. Divide into 4 bowls. Top each serving with banana, brown sugar, and chopped almonds (if desired).
6. Serve immediately.

Apple slices with peanut butter (Day 3)

Ingredients

- 2 medium apples, cored and sliced.
- 1/4 cup creamy peanut butter (natural or crunch), or to taste.

Directions

1. Place the apples in an airtight container and store them in the refrigerator until needed.
2. To make the filling, combine all of the ingredients in a food processor or blender and process until smooth and sticky, scraping down the sides as necessary.
3. Spoon ½ cup of filling onto each apple slice (5 to 6 slices per serving). Serve immediately

Breakfast muffin with eggs and vegetables (Day 4)

Ingredients

- 2 to 3 eggs, lightly beaten (preferred over the number one egg)
- 3-4 cups of baby spinach, chopped.
- 6 large mushrooms, sliced.
- 1/2 medium onion, diced.

- 1 teaspoon of nutmeg. (optional)
- Salt & pepper to taste.
- 3/4 cup of canned tomatoes, undrained and diced, or 1-2 fresh tomatoes thinly sliced (pitted and chopped).

Directions

1. Beat together ½ cup of egg and 3 tablespoons of water in a small bowl.
2. Coat the muffin pan with cooking spray, then make each muffin with a heaping tablespoonful of spinach, 1 mushroom, 1 tablespoon of onion; sprinkle with nutmeg and salt & pepper to taste.
3. Bake until the eggs are set (approximately 20 minutes at 350 F).
4. Cut muffins in half and serve with chopped tomatoes and egg mixture (like omelets)

Fruit Salad with Blueberries and Strawberries (Day 5)

Ingredients

- 1 cup blueberries
- 1 cup strawberries
- 2 tablespoons chopped fresh mint

- 1 teaspoon orange extract or 2 tablespoons fresh orange juice
- 1 tablespoon frozen orange juice concentrate
- ½ teaspoon ground cinnamon or apple pie spice (optional)
- Salt & pepper to taste.
- 1 cup of small seedless grapes, cut in half. (optional)

Directions

1. Combine the blueberries and strawberries in a medium bowl; sprinkle with mint, then drizzle with orange juice and add the other ingredients (except for the grapes). Mix gently until thoroughly combined. Add salt and pepper to taste.
2. Chill for up to 24 hours before serving, covered.
3. Serve the salad over crushed ice or refrigerate for up to 48 hours until you are ready to serve it.

Bread & butter (Day 6)

Ingredients

- 1 slice of bread.
- Butter, margarine, or spreads to taste.

Directions

1. Toast the bread lightly in the broiler or on a grill or stovetop grill pan.
2. Spread with butter and serve immediately.

Tuna Salad with Lemon (Day 7)

Ingredients

- 1 6-oz can of tuna, drained.
- 2 tablespoons chopped onion.
- ½ teaspoon lemon juice.
- ¼ cup of fat-free mayonnaise to taste 1/3 teaspoon of yellow mustard or vinegar. (optional)
- Salt & pepper to taste.

Directions

1. Pour the tuna into a large bowl.
2. Add the onion, lemon juice, mayonnaise, and salt & pepper to taste; stir gently. (optional)
3. Refrigerate until serving.

LUNCH RECIPES

Tuna salad with lettuce, cucumber, and tomato (Day 1)

Ingredients

- 1 cup of chopped cooked tuna, or skip this ingredient and use any other fish (preferred)
- 2 tablespoons of mayonnaise (preferred).
- 2 tablespoons sliced green onions.
- 2 tablespoons of tomato puree.
- 1 teaspoon of sweet pickle relish.
- Salt & pepper to taste.
- 3 cups lettuce, washed and torn into bite-sized pieces. (preferred) or 3 cups broccoli florets. (optional)
- 1 large cucumber, peeled and thinly sliced. (optional)

Directions

1. Combine the tuna, mayonnaise, green onions, and tomato puree in a medium bowl; stir until thoroughly combined.
2. Add salt and pepper to taste.
3. Add any of your favorite toppings (lettuce, cucumber, or tomato) to the tuna mixture to make a 1/2-finished salad that is ready for lunch or dinner. (optional)

Roasted veggie wrap with hummus (Day 2)

Ingredients

- 1 medium peeled and diced sweet potato
- ¼" slices (preferred over 1 medium zucchini).
- Salt & pepper to taste.
- 1 large or 2 small whole wheat tortillas
- 1 tablespoon hummus (preferred) or ½ avocado spread (optional)
- ½ cup shredded carrots. (optional)
- 1 tablespoon chopped fresh cilantro. (optional)

Directions

1. Put the harvested sweet potatoes and peppers into a large nonstick skillet over medium heat;

cover and cook 8–10 minutes until they are tender and browned on both sides, turning occasionally. Sprinkle with salt and pepper to taste.
2. Spread the hummus over half of the tortilla; add the vegetables, along with carrots and cilantro.
3. Fold the tortilla in half, wrap it in a paper towel, and microwave for approximately 30 seconds to 1 minute (add 30 seconds for each additional wrap).
4. Serve warm or at room temperature.

Grilled cheese sandwich with tomato soup (Day 3)

Ingredients

- Any type of low-fat cheese is available. (preferred)
- 2 slices whole wheat or rye bread (preferred).
- 1/2 cup tomato soup (optional)
- Salt & pepper to taste.

Directions

1. Preheat a nonstick skillet for 2 minutes.
2. Arrange the cheese slices in a single layer on one side of one slice of bread; top with the

other slice, turning it to completely cover the cheese.
3. Cook in the pan until both sides are golden brown; turn and cook an additional 5–10 seconds, so both sides are evenly golden brown.
4. Serve with soup or as desired (preferred).

Chicken salad with lettuce and corn (Day 4)

Ingredients

- 1 cup shredded cooked chicken (preferred) or tuna (optional)
- 2 tablespoons of mayonnaise (preferred).
- 1 tablespoon diced sweet pickle relish.
- 3 cups lettuce, washed & torn into bite-sized pieces. (Preferred) or 3 cups broccoli florets. (optional)

Directions

1. Combine the chicken, mayonnaise, and sweet pickle relish in a medium bowl; stir until thoroughly combined—season with salt and pepper to taste. Add any favorite toppings for lunch or dinner (lettuce or broccoli florets).
2. Serve over your choice of bread (white or whole wheat bread will absorb more of the dressing).

Snack: Granola bar with fruit (Day 5)

Ingredients

- 1–2 granola bars, any type. (preferred)
- 2 teaspoons dried fruit bits, such as chopped raisins, cranberries, and unsweetened coconut (optional)

Directions

1. Place the granola bars in a medium bowl; mix in the dried fruit until evenly distributed. Then pour in the milk and stir to evenly distribute the ingredients throughout the bar. Pack into an airtight container or bag and freeze up to 1 week before using.
2. Serve at room temperature.

Tuna melt (Day 6)

Ingredients

- 2 slices whole-wheat bread.
- 1/4 cup canned tuna, drained, or use cooked chicken, black beef beans (preferred).
- ¼ teaspoon salt & pepper to taste.

- 2 tablespoons mayonnaise or 2 tablespoons salsa or ¼ avocado spread (optional).
- 1 cup shredded cheddar cheese, divided between sandwiches. (preferred) or 4 servings of vegetables such as broccoli florets and carrots in any combination you like (optional).
- 1 tablespoon chopped fresh parsley if preferred.

Directions

1. Preheat the broiler.
2. Slice the bread into 1-inch slices.
3. Spread mayonnaise, tuna, salt, and pepper to taste on one slice of bread on a baking sheet, then top with cheese and whatever toppings you want (optional). Place under the broiler until the cheese has melted, then flip to brown both sides evenly. Replace the other slice of bread and repeat the process.
4. Serve at room temperature or chilled in a refrigerator container until needed for a midday snack or mid-afternoon lunch.

Tuna salad sandwich on whole-grain bread (Day 7)

Ingredients

- 2 slices of whole-wheat or rye bread.
- 1 water-packed tuna can, cooked chicken, or black beef beans (preferred).
- ½ avocado spread or 1 tablespoon mayonnaise (optional).
- ¼ teaspoon salt & pepper to taste.
- Lettuce leaf (optional) as garnish.

Directions

1. Add the lettuce and dressing to the tuna; mix well, stirring until thoroughly combined.
2. Serve in a lettuce leaf if you desire.
3. Serve chilled or at room temperature.

DINNER

Bean chili with cauliflower 'rice.' (Day 1)

Ingredients

- 1 cup canned black-eye or black beans, drained & rinsed (preferred), or cooked black beans.
- 1 cup chopped tomatoes, packed in their juice.

- ½ cup sliced green onions; ¼ cup olive oil (preferred) or 4 tablespoons of water.
- 2 cloves garlic, minced; ½ teaspoon salt & pepper to taste.
- ½ head cauliflower, cut into florets (optional)

Directions

1. In a nonstick saucepan, heat the oil or water with the onions and garlic. Saute until they're browned.
2. Add the tomatoes, beans, salt & pepper to taste, and 1½ cups of water; cover and simmer for about 30 minutes until all the liquid is evaporated. Stir occasionally to prevent from sticking (optional).
3. Add the cauliflower and cook until it softens.
4. Add some water if you need to thin out the chili with just a little bit of water to make it more sauce-like (preferred).
5. Serve in a bowl with a cup of steamed brown or white rice as a side dish (preferred).

Fried fish patties with spinach and mayonnaise (Day 2)

Ingredients

- One egg for coating, beaten.
- 2 slices whole-grain bread, cut into bite-sized pieces. (optional).
- Salt & pepper to taste.
- 1 teaspoon
- Worcestershire sauce.
- ½ medium red onion, sliced thinly
- 1 cup spinach
- ¼ cup chopped green onions. (optional)
- 2 tablespoons of mayonnaise (preferred).
- 1 scotch fillet or another firm white fish fillet, skinned & boned, and cut into bite-sized pieces or cubes (preferred) 4 ounces tofu, cubed (optional).

Directions

1. Spray an 8-inch or 9-inch nonstick skillet with nonstick cooking spray and heat to medium-high.
2. Add the bread pieces, place on the skillet, and cook, turning regularly, until golden brown.
3. Meanwhile, whisk the egg in a small bowl;

season with salt and pepper to taste; add mayonnaise and Worcestershire sauce; mix well.
4. Serve patties over spinach; top with onion slices, green onions, fried fish pieces or cubes, and mayonnaise mixture; serve immediately at room temperature.
5. Serve warm dishes at room temperature after heated or chilled in a refrigerator.
6. Serve with baked potatoes, large slices of sourdough bread, cornbread, polenta, or basmati rice (optional).

Chicken stir fry and soba noodles (Day 3)

Ingredients

- 1 cup cooked tofu (preferred) or pressed tofu, cubed.
- 1 tablespoon of soy sauce.
- 1 tablespoon of agave syrup (optional).
- 2 teaspoons toasted sesame oil.
- 2 cloves garlic, minced.
- ¼ medium onion, chopped finely.
- 1 teaspoon ginger, minced finely (optional).
- ½ head purple sprouting broccoli, chopped into bite-sized pieces (preferred) or ½ cup of green beans or pea pods. (optional).

- 1 teaspoon toasted sesame seeds (optional).

Directions

1. Cook the noodles.
2. Add the tofu, garlic, onion, and ginger; cook for about 5 minutes or until done.
3. Add the broccoli or green beans and cook for a further minute until tender but well coated with sauce. Serve warm dishes at room temperature after heated or chilled in a refrigerator container until needed.
4. Top with toasted sesame seeds; serve immediately at room temperature or chilled in a refrigerator container for an hour or two.

Tofu and squash burgers (Day 4)

Ingredients

- 1 cup of sliced mushrooms. (optional)
- ½ cup of chopped spinach, fresh or frozen. (optional)
- 1 teaspoon tamari soy sauce, shoyu soy sauce, or light soy sauce (preferred) or 1 teaspoon of balsamic vinegar. ½ teaspoon salt and pepper to taste
- 2 tablespoons lemon juice. (optional).

- 2 large portabella mushrooms, chopped finely (preferred). 4 ounces extra-firm tofu, pressed & crumbled into small pieces.
- 1/3 cup rolled oats.
- 1 tablespoon water.

Directions

1. Mix the mushrooms, spinach, and tamari in a bowl; season with salt and pepper to taste and add lemon juice if desired.
2. Sauté the mushroom mixture in a large skillet sprayed with nonstick spray until slightly tender; set aside for about 10 minutes before serving to allow flavors to meld.
3. In a large mixing bowl, mash the tofu, squash, oats, and water until well combined; season with salt and pepper to taste.
4. Shape into 3 patties and place on a skillet sprayed with nonstick spray; cook until done on each side, about 5 minutes per side. Serve warm dishes at room temperature after heated or chilled in a refrigerator container.

Curried chicken salad on crispbread or crackers (Day 5)

Ingredients

- 2 cups diced cooked chicken (preferred).
- 1 cup of chopped sweet potatoes (optional)
- 1½ cups of sliced mushrooms. (optional)
- Dried cranberries or raisins.
- ½ teaspoon salt and pepper to taste. (optional).
- 2 tablespoons sesame tahini. (preferred).
- 1 teaspoon curry powder.
- 1/8 teaspoon ground ginger (optional).

Directions

1. Mix the chicken, curry, cranberries/raisins, sweet potatoes if using, and seasonings together in a large bowl; cover and refrigerate for about an hour for flavors to meld together.
2. On a 1- to 2-inch layer of bread or cracker, spread the chicken salad; leave about ½-inch of bread or cracker on top.
3. Drizzle with tahini if desired and serve at room temperature or chilled in a refrigerator container for an hour or two to enjoy a morning meal.
4. Eat these crispy crispbreads for breakfast with

smoked salmon, eggs, and goat cheese on the side.
5. Serve as a finger food snack after being served at room temperature or chilled in a refrigerator container until needed.
6. Top with a dollop of yogurt, extra sesame tahini, or your favorite nut butter if you like these flat, round Scottish pancakes made from oats and wheat flour.

Curry chicken on rice (Day 6)

Ingredients

- 2 cups of cooked brown rice or basmati rice (preferred).
- 1 cup of sliced mushrooms. (optional)
- ½ cup of chopped spinach, fresh or frozen. (optional)
- 1 teaspoon tamari soy sauce. (optional).
- 1 tablespoon lemon juice. (optional)
- 2 tablespoons sesame tahini. (preferred).
- 1 teaspoon curry powder.
- ½ teaspoon salt and pepper to taste.

Directions

1. Cook and add salt to the rice in a large saucepan sprayed with nonstick spray; cook for 20 minutes, covered, or until done.
2. Open the saucepan and stir the rice, mushrooms, spinach/sweet potatoes if using, curry powder, tahini, lemon juice if desired, & salt and pepper to taste; cover and cook for an additional 5 minutes.
3. Serve warm dishes at room temperature or chilled in a refrigerator container after heated or cooled down.
4. Top with your favorite ketchup for a hearty eggs benedict breakfast.
5. Serve after heated or cooled down at room temperature or chilled in a refrigerator container until needed.
6. Top with a dollop of yogurt, extra sesame tahini, or your favorite nut butter if you like these flat, round Scottish pancakes made from oats and wheat flour.

Crab cakes and avocado salsa on an Israeli couscous salad (Day 7)

Ingredients

- 1 cup cooked harissa bel poushki rice
- 2 teaspoons of salt and pepper to taste.
- 8 ounces of lump crab meat (preferred) or 1 pound of fresh crab meat, cleaned and picked over.
- 1 medium shallot, minced.
- 4 ounces extra-firm tofu, pressed & crumbled into small pieces.
- ¼ cup toasted sesame seeds (optional).
- 2 cloves garlic, minced.
- 1 teaspoon ginger, minced finely (optional).
- 1 teaspoon ground cumin.
- ¼ cup lemon juice.
- 12 cup freshly chopped parsley or cilantro, to taste
- ½ head of red cabbage, chopped into bite-sized pieces. (optional)
- 1 tablespoon tamari soy sauce, shoyu soy sauce, nori flakes, or sea salt & pepper to taste (optional).
- 1 cup of finely chopped fresh mangoes or pears (optional).
- 1 cup of chopped pineapple or apples (optional)

Directions

1. Place the tofu in a large mixing bowl, crumble and mash with a fork until the texture resembles ground meat; season with salt and pepper.
2. Set aside for about 10 minutes. In a mixing bowl, combine the cabbage, tofu, crab meat, and remaining ingredients (except garnishes) in a small saucepan sprayed with nonstick spray; cook, covered, until tender, 5 minutes; set aside to cool slightly before adding to the tofu mixture, crab meat, and remaining ingredients (except garnishes); mix well but gently.
3. In a large skillet sprayed with nonstick spray, cook the onion until translucent; add garlic, ginger, cumin, and lemon juice; cook and stir until fragrant, about 1 minute.
4. Add the crab mixture to the onion mixture and fold in gently until well combined. The final product should be crumbly but not a wet mess. If it is too wet, add some of the drained rice to thicken as desired; mix well with your hands by rotating your hands all around in a figure-eight motion to blend flavors.
5. Spray another skillet with nonstick spray; cook crab cake mixture on each side until browned,

about 3 minutes per side. Serve warm dishes at room temperature after heated or chilled in a refrigerator container for an hour or two to enjoy a morning meal.

SNACKS

Whole grain rice cake with nut butter (Day 1)

Ingredients

- 1 cup of rice cakes. (optional).
- ½ cup of your favorite nut butter.

Directions

1. Spread the nut butter on a rice cake and enjoy it at room temperature, or chill it in a refrigerator container until you're ready to eat this snack that you can make at home!

Sweet toasted oat cereal with dried cranberries (Day 2)

Ingredients

- ½ cup plain yogurt with favorite toppings. (optional)

- 1/3 cup whole-grain cereal, oats, and wheat flakes or ½ slice of bread (optional).
- 2 tablespoons dried fruit, raisins preferred (optional).

Directions

1. Rinse the cereal in a bowl of water; drain and place the cereal in a saucepan sprayed with nonstick spray, and sauté until lightly browned.
2. Add the raisins and heat for a minute more; add the yogurt or toppings if desired.

Crispy baked muffin top croutons (Day 3)

Ingredients

- 2 tablespoons sesame seeds or other seeds of choice (optional)
- 1 cup of croutons or bread cracker (optional).
- 1 tablespoon melted butter. (optional)

Directions

1. Spray a baking sheet sprayed with nonstick spray; add the seeds and cook until lightly browned.
2. Add the bread or crouton pieces and melt the

butter if using; remove from oven and cool slightly before serving on top of your favorite vegetables, soups, salads, or tofu salads.
3. Top with your favorite ketchup for a hearty eggs benedict breakfast.

Crispy flatbread with hummus (Day 4)

Ingredients

- 1 whole-grain flatbread or other whole-grain bread.

Directions

1. Spread the bottom of the bread with the hummus, if preferred, and top with your favorite sliced veggie and seed mixture of choice; drizzle with fat-free vegetable broth or a low-fat soy sauce if desired.
2. Heat in a toaster for about 5 minutes or in an oven until crispy; serve warm dishes at room temperature or chilled in a refrigerator container after heated or cooled down.

Cocoa protein ball (Day 5)

Ingredients

- 2 tablespoons unsweetened cocoa powder. (optional)
- 1 tablespoon of peanut butter. (optional)
- 1 teaspoon of honey.

Directions

1. Mix the cocoa powder and honey in a pan sprayed with nonstick spray; heat until a ball forms from the mixture.
2. Spoon the peanut butter on the ball and roll it into a ball to just above the size of a coin; serve with your favorite berries or a banana.

Quick breakfast muffin (Day 6)

Ingredients

- 1 ½ cups old-fashioned oatmeal rolled oats or regular whole-wheat flour. 1 egg, beaten.
- ½ cup low-fat yogurt or cottage cheese.
- 2 teaspoons wheat germ, flax seeds, or your favorite nut butter.
- ¼ teaspoon vanilla extract.

Directions

1. Preheat a toaster oven or a medium-sized oven.
2. Mix the oatmeal, egg, yogurt, wheat germ, and vanilla if desired; make reservations and pour into muffin tin.
3. Bake for 10 to 15 minutes at 350 degrees F (175 degrees C) until done, or serve warm at room temperature or chilled in a refrigerator container after heating or cooling.

Oven bagel (Day 7)

Ingredients

- 2 cups of oats, cooked.
- ½ cup of chopped walnut pieces. (optional)
- 1 egg white, beaten.
- Pinch salt and pepper to taste.

Directions

1. Combine the oats and egg white in a large bowl; stir well to combine; mix the walnut pieces if desired; sprinkle with the salt and pepper and place inside an oven bag or a large zipper-lock bag; seal the bag or place it in a large zipper-lock bag with a clean kitchen towel on top, and

put it in the preheated oven at 350 degrees F (175 degrees C).
2. Cook for about 20 minutes or until done; serve warm dishes at room temperature or chilled in a refrigerator container after heated or cooled down.
3. Enjoy with your favorite ketchup for a hearty eggs benedict breakfast.

WHAT THE RESEARCH SAYS

Trusted Source investigated the best dietary approach for effective and long-term weight loss in people who are overweight or obese in a review published in 2018. The study concluded that there is no one-size-fits-all diet and that individualization is the best approach to helping people lose weight effectively and long-term. The most successful diets used a variety of diet plans, each with its benefits, instead of just one diet that was the standard. The researchers found that the best weight-loss diets combined low-fat and high-carbohydrate diets.

It is important to note that this research review considered only short-term (less than 12 weeks) evidence on the weight loss effects of the most popular diets. More long-term studies may be needed to determine which diet is best for maintaining long-term weight control or to find the optimal diet approach for long-term weight maintenance in overweight individuals.

In addition, this review did not include any studies on exercise and dietary patterns.

In the same review, the importance of the following approaches for weight loss is emphasized:

- Avoiding added sugars
- Limiting processed foods
- Consuming whole grain products
- Consuming more fruits and vegetables
- Consuming whole foods
- Eating whole food
- Eating a low-fat diet
- Avoiding too much alcohol
- Not dieting and then overeating.

Tips on how to lose weight with a balanced diet

When you're trying to lose weight and get healthy, you can make it easier for yourself by following this diet:

- Include heart-healthy foods in your diet.
- Consume foods that are beneficial to your brain.
- Planning meals and snacks and only buying what's on the grocery list

- Understanding portion sizes and macronutrient ratios
- Including protein and fiber in every meal
- Experimenting with new herbs and spices to add variety to meals and reduce the need for extra sugar, salt, and fat
- Batch-cooking healthy meals for the freezer
- Avoiding long periods without food to avoid cravings for unhealthy snacks
- Teaming up with a friend who can help you stick to a diet and exercise routine.
- A trusted source of moderate-intensity physical activity on most or all days of the week
- A balanced breakfast for weight loss and maintenance

While it is preferable to consume all the nutrients you need from actual food, vitamins and minerals can be found in pills, powders, liquids, and sprays. Supplements are not a substitute for food; they should be taken only when appropriate based on the dietary needs of an individual patient or care recipient. Unsafe supplements should be avoided by people with low bone density or other medical conditions. Weight loss that is healthy is not a quick fix. It takes time, patience, commitment, and the ability to sustain good habits for life.

5

BODY FAT PERCENTAGE AND IDEAL WEIGHT CHART, BMI CALCULATOR

The body mass index (BMI) measures body fat that applies to adult men and women and is based on height and weight. There are different ways to calculate the BMI, with a simpler version using just weight in kilograms (kg).

OVERWEIGHT, OBESITY, AND BODY FAT

Body fat is the main factor in the increase of your weight. For this reason, we need to know your percentage of body fat so that we can get a better estimate of your ideal weight. The healthiest and safest weight is that you can maintain without any excess weight. Adipose tissue performs a variety of vital functions. Its primary function is to store lipids, which the body uses to generate energy. It also secretes several important hormones and provides cushioning and insulation to the body.

The two types of fat in the body are essential and storage fat. The term "essential body fat" refers to a type of fat that is found in nearly every part of the body. Essential fat levels differ between men and women, with men having around 2-5 percent and women having around 10-13 percent. Men's healthy body fat levels are typically 8-19%, while women's healthy body fat levels are 21-33 percent. While having too much body fat can be harmful to one's health, having too little body fat can also be harmful. A medical professional should discuss maintaining a body fat percentage below or within the essential body fat percentage range.

Storage fat, also known as "body fat," is fat that accumulates in adipose tissue, whether it's subcutaneous fat (found deep beneath the dermis and wrapped around vital organs) or visceral fat (found inside the abdominal cavity, between organs). While some storage fat is beneficial, excessive amounts can have serious health consequences.

Because insufficient measures are taken to curb increasing body fat, excess body fat leads to being overweight and eventually to obesity. It's important to remember that being overweight doesn't always mean you have a lot of fat on your body. The composition of a person's body weight includes (but is not limited to) body fat, muscle, bone density, and water content. As a result, extremely muscular people are frequently labeled as obese.

The rate at which body fat accumulates varies from person to person and is influenced by various factors, including genetics and behavioral factors such as inactivity and overeating. Certain people may find it more difficult to lose body fat stored in the abdominal region due to various factors. On the other hand, diet and exercise management have been shown to help people lose weight. It's important to keep in mind that men and women store body fat differently, and this can change over time. Excess body fat can develop around the stomach in men and the buttocks and thighs in women after the age of 40 as a result of decreased sexual hormones (or after menopause in some cases for women).

Body fat is critical for normal body function, but an excess can be dangerous. Too little body fat can also lead to various health problems. With that in mind, the following information will help you understand your body fat percentage and its effect on your health.

HOW MUCH BODY FAT PERCENTAGE IS TOO MUCH?

To determine your body fat percentage, you'll need a calculator and a tape measure or a hanging scale (which measures BMI). Here's how to calculate it:

Total body fat = weight in pounds x [body fat percentage x 703].

Age (Years)	Body Fat Percentage (%)	
	Men	Women
20	8.5%	17.7%
25	10.5%	18.4%
30	12.7%	19.3%
35	13.7%	21.5%
40	15.3%	22.2%
45	16.4%	22.9%
50	18.9%	25.2%
55	20.9%	26.3%

References; Jackson AS, Pollock ML. Generalized equations for predicting body density of men. Br J Nutr. 1978;40(3):497-504
Jackson AS. Pollock ML. Ward A. Generalized equations for predicfing body density of women. Med Sci Sports Exerc. 1980:12(3):175-81

If you want to be healthy and fit, then the ideal body fat percentage for a woman is between 21 and 33 percent, while a man's healthy range is between 8 and 19 percent. Each person has different body fat goals depending on their health, age, and fitness requirements. If you're trying to improve your overall health or lose weight, aim for the ideal body fat range. Bodybuilders (who are more often men) have higher goals for body fat percentage because they need more lean muscle mass to be successful in their sport.

WHAT SHOULD YOU DO IF YOU FALL OUTSIDE OF THOSE RANGES?

The body fat ranges discussed here are ideal for overall health and fitness. If you fall outside of this range, speak with your doctor about the best course of action for you. While it is important to maintain a healthy weight for overall health and fitness, your body fat percentage has a greater impact on your health. This is especially true for those who are considered obese and overweight.

The difference between being healthy and unhealthy based on body fat is likely to be less than the difference between being skinny to obese. This is because the majority of the body's functional organs are located within fat. Some people struggle to accept that there is a significant difference between being healthy and fit and being unhealthy. It's important to remember, though, that health problems aren't always obvious.

In fact, many of the health problems we experience today were not on display until recently because they're often associated with other risk factors that are also associated with other risk factors.

An individual's ideal weight can be defined as making them feel the most at ease.

Maintaining a healthy weight, on the other hand, can lower a person's risk of developing a variety of health problems, including:

- Cancer
- Heart disease
- Diabetes
- High blood pressure
- Stroke
- Obesity
- Osteoarthritis
- Reduced glucose tolerance by 20%
- Reduced life expectancy of 10 years

The body mass index (BMI) is a simple number calculated from an individual's weight and height. It has been used as a reliable indicator of body fatness for decades.

Body mass index (BMI) estimates total body fat based on height and weight that applies to adult men and women. BMI does not measure the percentage of body fat, but it's been shown to be a good indicator of health risks associated with various levels of body fatness. Since BMI doesn't measure body fat percentage, you should use it as one tool among many when assessing your overall health risks.

BMI is an inexpensive and simple way to screen for weight categories that may lead to health problems. It's not a diagnostic tool, though; it simply indicates whether weight might be a health concern.

However, not everyone who is overweight will experience health problems. However, while the extra weight may not be affecting health right now, researchers believe that weight management issues could cause problems in the future.

The Body Mass Index (BMI) is a common tool for calculating a person's weight about their height. A BMI calculation yields a single number classified into the following groups.

BMI in Adults	Weight Status
<18.5	Underweight
18.5–24.9	Normal
25.0–29.9	Overweight
>30.0	Obese

What is the formula for calculating BMI?

Imperial English Formula

Weight (lbs) x 703 ÷ Height (inch^2)

Metric BMI Formula

Weight (kg) / Height (m^2)

WHO WOULDN'T BENEFIT FROM USING A BMI CALCULATOR?

Muscle builders, long-distance runners, pregnant women, the elderly, and young children are not eligible for BMI. The BMI does not consider whether the weight is carried as muscle or fat; only the number is taken into account. Athletes, for example, may have a higher BMI but are not at a higher risk of developing health problems. A lower BMI is associated with less muscle mass, such as in children who have not finished growing or the elderly who may be losing muscle mass. BMI is ineffective because a woman's body composition changes during pregnancy and lactation.

BMI calculator for obese and overweight people:

The BMI is an impractical method for identifying whether someone is overweight or obese because it does not consider the level of muscle mass. In addition, BMI doesn't consider racial differences in weight status. However, BMI can be useful to health professionals trying to judge whether an individual may have a weight problem.

A simple formula can help determine if you are underweight, at risk of being underweight, or overweight.

Who wouldn't benefit from using a BMI calculator?

Muscle builders, long-distance runners, pregnant women, the elderly, and young children are not eligible for BMI. The BMI does not consider whether the weight is muscle or fat; it only considers the numerical value. Individuals with increased muscle mass, such as athletes, may have a higher BMI but are not at an increased risk of developing health problems. A lower BMI is associated with less muscle mass, such as in children who have not reached their full growth potential or the elderly who are losing muscle mass. Because a woman's body composition changes during pregnancy and lactation, BMI is ineffective.

GUIDELINE FOR WEIGHT AND HEIGHT

The BMI tables from the National Institutes of Health (NIH) Trusted Source are used in the following weight and height chart to determine how much a person's weight should be for their height.

Height	Normal weight BMI 19–24	Overweight BMI 25–29	Obesity BMI 30–39	Severe obesity BMI 40+
4 ft. 10 in (58 in)	91–115 lb.	119–138 lb.	143–186 lb.	191–258 lb.
4 ft. 11 in (59 in)	94–119 lb.	124–143 lb.	148–193 lb.	198–267 lb.
5ft (60 in")	97–123 lb.	128–148 lb.	153–199 lb.	204–276 lb.
5 ft. 1 in (61 in)	100–127 lb.	132–153 lb.	158–206 lb.	211–285 lb.
5 ft. 2 in (62 in)	104–131 lb.	136–158 lb.	164–213 lb.	218–295 lb.
5 ft. 3 in (63 in)	107–135 lb.	141–163 lb.	169–220 lb.	225–304 lb.
5 ft. 4 in (64 in)	110–140 lb.	145–169 lb.	174–227 lb.	232–314 lb.
5 ft. 5 in (65 in)	114–144 lb.	150–174 lb.	180–234 lb.	240–324 lb.

Height				
5 ft. 6 in (66 in)	118–148 lb.	155–179 lb.	186–241 lb.	247–334 lb.
5 ft. 7 in (67 in)	121–153 lb.	159–185 lb.	191–249 lb.	255–344 lb.
5 ft. 8 in (68 in)	125–158 lb.	164–190 lb.	197–256 lb.	262–354 lb.
5 ft. 9 in (69 in)	128–162 lb.	169–196 lb.	203–263 lb.	270–365 lb.
5 ft. 10 in (70 in)	132–167 lb.	174–202 lb.	209–271 lb.	278–376 lb.
5 ft. 11 in (71 in)	136–172 lb.	179–208 lb.	215–279 lb.	286–386 lb.
6 ft. (72 in)	140–177 lb.	184–213 lb.	221–287 lb.	294–397 lb.
6 ft. 1 in (73 in)	144–182 lb.	189–219 lb.	227–295 lb.	302–408 lb.
6 ft. 2 in (74 in)	148–186 lb.	194–225 lb.	233–303 lb.	311–420 lb.
6 ft. 3 in (75 in)	152–192 lb.	200–232 lb.	240–311 lb.	319–431 lb.
6 ft. 4 in (76 in)	156–197 lb.	205–238 lb.	246–320 lb.	328–443 lb.

Calculate your BMI using the following calculator. It is only to be used as a guide and not for diagnostic or therapeutic purposes.

BMI calculation is limited to age and gender only. The BMI chart can be used from 18 to 70 years old, and it only goes up to 85 years old. The BMI calculation will not give you the correct result if you are older than 85 years old; this will result in an underestimated BMI.

BMI was first calculated in the 1920s and is still used today. It has been adopted by government agencies and medical associations to determine health risks and recommended weight ranges. BMI is also used in occupational health and at some universities to determine a person's eligibility for participation in sports. BMI was originally developed by French railroad engineer and anthropologist Adolphe Quetelet.

The research found that women with the highest total body fat (a risk factor for cardiovascular disease) were 43 percent less likely to be obese than those with the lowest body fat. This study also demonstrated a significant relationship between visceral fat and waist circumference. A person's body mass index is a good indicator of their overall risk for health problems associated with high body fat levels.

WHAT IS CHOLESTEROL? WAYS TO LOWER YOUR CHOLESTEROL

We want to lose weight first when we decide to change our lifestyle. What about cholesterol, though? There is mixed information on how much cholesterol you need or should have, so it can be hard to know where to start. You may also be wondering if there are any ways to lower your cholesterol without becoming overweight or changing your lifestyle. Cholesterol has indeed gotten a bad reputation over the years, but it is an essential part of your body's function.

THE FACTS

Cholesterol itself is not fat. It isn't saturated or unsaturated. Cholesterol is a type of lipid that helps build your cell membranes and many other parts of your body like hormones, vitamin D, and bile acids to help you digest food. However, when we think of cholesterol and how it affects our health, we're referring to the ratio of high-density lipoprotein (HDL) to low-density lipoprotein (LDL) that it contains.

The term "good cholesterol" refers to HDL, which aids the body in removing excess fat. LDL is the 'bad cholesterol because it stores fat. Your body needs some LDL to build cell walls, but too much leads to clogged arteries and heart disease.

When trying to lose weight and lower your cholesterol, you need to remember that fat in food doesn't raise your cholesterol levels unless they are saturated or trans fats. Cholesterol itself doesn't cause high blood pressure or heart disease either. The unhealthy lifestyle choices around eating too many saturated fats and not getting enough potassium, fiber, and other nutrients can help lower cholesterol levels.

Reducing your cholesterol level naturally

Did you know that for every 10% reduction in your cholesterol level, your risk of a heart attack drops by 20% to 30%? There's even more good news: most of us can lower our cholesterol naturally, without the use of medications. Simple lifestyle changes, especially for those with high cholesterol levels, can have a significant impact on lowering cholesterol.

The most effective methods for altering one's lifestyle to affect cholesterol levels positively are:

1. Fruits, vegetables, whole grains, and beans should be prioritized.

To lower our cholesterol levels, we don't have to become vegetarians. Still, the more vegetables, fruits, potatoes, and other naturally fiber-rich plant foods we consume, the healthier we will be. These foods have proven to lower cholesterol levels naturally and reduce the risk of heart disease.

2. Exercise is also a healthy lifestyle choice

It helps increase the number of HDL cholesterol and reduce the amount of LDL. Exercise benefits your heart by lowering cholesterol levels and improving blood flow.

3. Keep an eye on your fat intake

Learn about the "bad" fats to avoid and the "good" fats to limit or increase. At all costs, saturated and trans fats should be avoided. While plant-based fats effectively lower LDL cholesterol, they are ineffective at lowering total cholesterol.

At the same time, try to increase your healthy fat intake to make up for fats you are avoiding. The healthier your fat intake is, the better your cholesterol levels and metabolism.

4. Drink plenty of water

The amount of water we consume directly affects our cholesterol levels. Drinking enough water helps the liver remove potentially unhealthy cholesterol content. If you are dehydrated, the liver will produce more cholesterol. Because most of our bodies are water, you'll need to increase your water intake. If you drink too much water at a time, it's recommended that you 'go back to the drawing board' and start with replacing only half of what you are taking in by drinking water. The daily requirement of water is 8-10 glasses.

5. Stay away from cigarettes and excessive alcohol

Smoking raises your bad cholesterol level and increases the risk of lung cancer, heart disease, and stroke. Excessive drinking can lead to more high-calorie eating, which can raise your cholesterol levels even more. Alcohol also depletes your body with vitamin B-6 and Folate, which are important in lowering the risk of heart disease. Alcohol is also not good for you when trying to lose weight.

6. Talk to your doctor about medications to treat high cholesterol

Medications are available for those who want to lower their cholesterol levels, but medications aren't the end-all solution. They can have side effects and may be more beneficial than others. For example, women who take statins and experience memory loss, headaches, or joint pain might consider lowering their intake or looking at natural alternatives such as fish oil instead. Always be sure that you are within a normal range before starting a medication.

Lowering your cholesterol naturally can effectively prevent heart disease risk factors without the side effects of medications or the strain of making major lifestyle changes. You can even lower your cholesterol with just a few changes to your diet and exercise schedule.

ESSENTIAL NUTRIENTS THAT HELP IMPROVE CHOLESTEROL LEVELS

Vitamin B-6

A deficiency in this B vitamin increases the risk of cardiovascular diseases by 25% and increases the risk of colon cancer by 40%. It's required for the breakdown of carbohydrates, fats, and proteins.

Folic acid

This B vitamin is needed to maintain the upper levels of the genetic material DNA and RNA. If this vital component is deficient, it could lead to deficiency in other B vitamins. The recommended folic acid intake is 400 mcg per day for women, which can be increased if taking drug-based preparations for birth control or other medical reasons.

Magnesium

Magnesium plays a vital role as an active ingredient in more than 300 enzyme reactions in your body. It is necessary for the disposal of glucose out of the cells and is also needed for energy metabolism, maintenance of the bone structure, and transmission of nerve impulses.

Potassium

It plays an important role as an electrolyte in energy metabolism and blood pressure regulation, particularly important in your heart muscle. A deficiency could cause cardiac arrhythmias and sudden death. Adults should consume 4 to 6 servings of potassium-rich foods per day, including fruits, vegetables, low-fat dairy, or meat.

Vitamin D

This vitamin is needed to maintain a physiological balance by regulating calcium absorption in your body and maintaining the mineral content in bones. It also is essential for maintaining healthy teeth and bones. Skin exposure to sunlight improves the body's ability to metabolize vitamin D from your diet and foods such as salmon, tuna, and mushrooms. You can also obtain vitamin D-fortified foods such as milk, orange juice, and certain margarine products.

Vitamin E

It's required for red blood cells to function properly. Vitamin E works in combination with fats to help lower cholesterol levels by improving fat metabolism. This nutrient also helps fight against the damage of cell membranes and improves the stability of cell membranes by promoting their ability to retain nutrients. Vitamin E should be consumed with other antioxidants like vitamin C, selenium, and zinc.

Zinc

It is needed for fertility, immune function, and the adequate development of your sexual organs. It also helps with carbohydrate, protein, and fat metabolism. Zinc works with vitamin A and antioxidant enzymes to protect against free radicals that can damage cholesterol levels and other cell structures.

Fiber

It is a critical nutrient for lowering cholesterol. It helps you maintain a healthy weight, lower cholesterol levels, decrease the risk of heart disease by lowering blood pressure, help lower LDL and triglyceride levels, and help improve your digestive health. You can increase your intake of this nutrient by eating more fruits, vegetables, whole-grain cereals, beans, peas, lentils, or brown rice. Always drink enough fluids when consuming high-fiber foods to maintain proper hydration in your body.

Magnesium citrate

This form of magnesium can help improve cholesterol levels by improving blood glucose levels. It also helps maintain normal blood pressure, reduce triglyceride levels, stabilize heart rhythm and regulate nerve transmission. You can also take this supplement as a part of your healthy lifestyle.

Chlorophyll

It works together with other nutrients like proteins, minerals, vitamins, and trace elements like zinc in the human body to remove toxins from the bloodstream and maintain a balanced environment within your cells. Additionally, it aids in the fight against free radicals, which can cause the body's cholesterol levels to rise. You can take chlorophyll as a part of your daily supplement routine or include it during food preparation to improve its color and flavor.

Fish oil

This supplement is often recommended to improve cholesterol levels. It's necessary to keep your skin, hair, and nails in good shape. It also works as an anti-inflammatory that combats against asthma, arthritis, cancer, and heart disease. Be sure to take a supplement that is higher in omega -3 fatty acids than omega -6 fatty acids.

Other supplements

B vitamins are needed in the diet to help convert food into energy. They help regulate cholesterol levels, prevent heart disease and keep your nervous system working properly. If you can not get enough of these vitamins from food sources such as legumes, vegetables, and whole grains, you can supplement your diet with a B vitamin supplement.

Taking care of your cholesterol levels is essential to protect your heart and overall health. Losing weight and getting more exercise can be challenging for you. However, when you make these necessary changes with the help of a medical practitioner and include supplements to achieve your wellness goals, you will see that your cholesterol levels are better than before.

HEALTH BENEFITS OF YOGA

Yoga plays an important role for many people in the world today. It is a way for people to improve their lifestyle and overall health.

Yoga can help you in a variety of ways, including:

Improving heart health

Exercises such as yoga reduce your blood pressure and help lower cholesterol levels.

Reducing stress

Different forms of yoga, such as kundalini, are a great way to quiet your mind and relax after a long day at work.

Improving flexibility

Practicing yoga can keep you limber even if you are not very active throughout the week. You will enjoy your activities even more, when you have increased flexibility in your joints.

Increasing energy levels

As you stand or lie down, it seems like it would be easy to relax and fall asleep during a yoga session. However, this is not what happens when people practice regularly. After a few sessions, they feel more energized and clearheaded than they did before beginning yoga.

Preventing diseases

Regular yoga can help prevent osteoporosis by strengthening your muscles, joints, and bones. It also helps prevent the onset of other diseases such as diabetes and cancer.

Improving sleep

As time goes on, life gets busier for many people. A lack of sleep can lead to problems such as an increased risk of heart disease and depression. As you practice yoga regularly, you will likely notice that you fall asleep quicker and stay peacefully asleep throughout the night than you did before you began practicing.

Improving mental health

As you practice yoga, you will feel more relaxed, focused, and positive throughout the day. Regular yoga practice can also improve your mental health and prevent the onset of mental disorders, in addition to the benefits already mentioned.

Preventing joint problems

When you practice yoga, you will notice that your joints improve over time.

Yoga sessions can help you achieve a better posture and make it easier to move around without pain or stiffness in your joints.

Protecting against stroke

A yoga session can help reduce the risk of a stroke by improving your blood pressure, which helps keep your blood vessels from narrowing and increasing blood flow to the brain. Regular yoga sessions can also help lower stress levels, known as "stress reduction." The combination of these three things helps protect against a stroke.

Improving balance

Regular yoga practice can improve your balance, walking, and standing skills. By improving your balance, you will have better control and coordination over other parts of your body.

Improving digestion

Yoga can help your digestion if you practice it on a regular basis. This is because yoga helps strengthen the digestive organs, which can improve digestion efficiency. It also helps keep you regular and eliminate constipation.

Decreasing aging

Yoga practices such as Ashtanga and Kundalini yoga are a great way to prevent yourself from aging too quickly. These particular yoga practices help keep you young and healthy by promoting circulation, keeping your mind focused, improving flexibility and balance, reducing stress levels, and staying limber.

Keeping your skin healthy

Suppose you have ever practiced yoga with a traditional guru in India or elsewhere. In that case, you will likely remember that they used to encourage you to practice specific poses that would clear up your skin. Even if your body doesn't necessarily suffer from acne or pimples while practicing yoga, it is still a good idea to regularly do poses that strengthen the skin and promote blood flow through the body. This will help improve your skin's overall health.

Improving your reproductive health

Yoga is an excellent way to improve the overall health of your reproductive system, which can help you become more fertile and pregnant. Practicing yoga regularly can help you have strong pelvic floor muscles, which are sensitive to estrogen and progesterone levels in the body. This can improve ovulation, menstruation, and even menopause symptoms such as hot flashes.

HOW DOES YOGA HELP WITH WEIGHT LOSS?

Everyone knows that exercise is important for weight loss, but it's not for everyone. Yoga is a great activity that many people like to incorporate into their weekly routine, as it helps tone muscles and increases flexibility. While weight loss is not the primary benefit of yoga, it can still assist you in meeting your weight loss objectives in other ways. Regular yoga practice is a great way to lose weight naturally. It may be more effective than other forms of exercise, such as cycling or running, because it is low-impact and suitable for overweight people.

Yoga can assist with weight loss in a variety of ways. It can help you relax and focus on breathing, which helps you release endorphins and relax your mind. When you can relax, it becomes easier to shed stubborn pounds and make it easier for you to stay focused on losing weight instead of turning back to unhealthy habits. Yoga can also reduce stress levels, which is another common reason people gain weight.

Yoga can also improve your overall health, which provides more benefits than simply a slimmer body. Practicing yoga regularly will improve your digestion system and strengthen your immune system, so you are less likely to get sick and have to stay home from work or cancel a workout session. Yoga can also help you stay limber and flexibly, which will provide many other benefits, such as improving athletic performance.

Yoga's detoxifying effects are a pretty common topic of discussion among people who practice it. The benefits of a detoxification program are not just about losing weight. A new day-to-day lifestyle that involves healthy eating, regular exercise, and a measure of detoxification can have many health benefits, even if it does not improve your weight or make you lose weight quickly.

Yoga and calorie expenditure

While yoga isn't traditionally thought of as a cardiovascular workout, some poses are more physically demanding than others.

Yoga styles that are active and intense help you burn the most calories. This could help you avoid gaining weight. More physical yoga styles include ashtanga, vinyasa, and power yoga.

Hot yoga studios typically offer vinyasa and power yoga. These types of yoga keep you moving almost continuously, which aids in calorie burning.

Yoga may also aid in developing muscle tone and the improvement of your metabolism.

While restorative yoga isn't a particularly physically demanding form, it can still aid in weight loss. In one study, restorative yoga was found to be effective in helping overweight women lose weight, including abdominal fat.

These findings are particularly encouraging for people whose weight makes more vigorous yoga difficult.

By burning calories, increasing mindfulness, and reducing stress, yoga may be a promising way to help with behavioral change, weight loss, and maintenance. These factors may assist you in reducing your food intake and becoming more aware of the negative consequences of overeating.

Consider how you'll feel about yourself once you've shed some pounds.

1. Will you be proud of your new figure?
2. Will you be more confident and self-assured?
3. Is the scale going to be your number one motivator to stay on track?
4. Or will you rely on your peer pressure and social media to keep up appearances?
5. When it comes down to it, what kind of weight loss do you want: a physical change or a change in how others see you and treat you?

WHEN IT COMES TO LOSING WEIGHT, HOW OFTEN SHOULD YOU PRACTICE YOGA?

Yoga should be practiced as frequently as possible to aid in weight loss. Three to five times per week, you can do a more active, intense practice for at least an hour.

Balance your practice with a more gentle, relaxing class on alternate days.

If you're a beginner, begin with a 20-minute practice and work your way up. This enables you to increase your strength and flexibility while avoiding injuries. Each week, allow yourself one full day of rest before you begin to practice again.

If you're an experienced yogi, choose a different style each time you assess your body and needs. Don't get stuck on a certain style, and don't stick with the same thing too long. To reap the benefits of yoga and keep yourself interested in it, attend as many classes as you can.

Injury prevention is another factor that will play a role in determining how often to practice yoga. If you have an existing injury or chronic pain, don't overdo it on one day or strain yourself too much with the poses. As with any exercise, listen to your body and make adjustments where necessary.

Combine your yoga practice with cardiovascular activities such as walking, cycling, or swimming to maximize your results.

POSES TO PRACTICE AT HOME

Try these at-home poses if you don't have time for a full yoga session.

Sun Salutations

Perform a minimum of ten Sun Salutations. Increase the intensity by holding certain positions for longer periods or accelerating the pace.

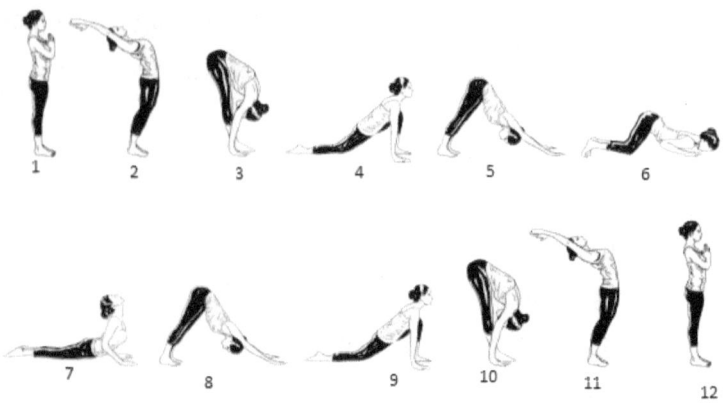

1. Inhale as you raise your arms overhead from a standing position.
2. As you swan dive into a Forward Bend, exhale.
3. Reintroduce the Plank pose by leaping, stepping, or walking your feet back into the Plank pose.
4. Maintain this position for a minimum of five breaths.
5. Bend your knees and squat to the floor.
6. Extend your legs, face the mat with the tops of your feet, and place your hands beneath your shoulders.
7. Inhale to lift into Cobra pose partially, halfway, or completely.
8. Exhale to return to the starting position and press into Downward Facing Dog.

9. Maintain this pose for a minimum of five breaths.
10. Exhale as you leap, step, or walk your feet to the mat's top and stand in a Forward Bend.
11. Inhale, then raise your arms overhead.
12. Exhale to bring your arms back into contact with your body.

Boat pose

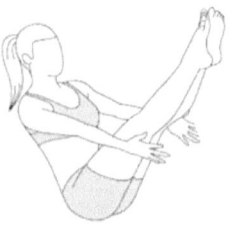

This pose engages your entire body, particularly your core, and assists in stress reduction.

1. Sit on the floor, legs straight ahead. Place your hands on the floor behind your hips.
2. Lift through the top of your sternum and lean back slightly, but don't round your back. Weigh evenly between your tripod and tailbone.

3. Inhale deeply and bend your knees. Lift your thighs to a 45-degree angle above the floor while keeping your knees bent.
4. Slowly straighten your knees, raising your toes slightly above the level of your eyes if possible. If this isn't possible, keep your knees bent and your shins parallel to the floor.
5. Draw your shoulders back and extend both arms forward alongside the legs, parallel to the floor, palms facing in, while keeping your heart open and spine long. Maintain a flat, firm lower belly that isn't hard or thick.
6. Breathe while pointing your toes or flexing your heels. At first, try holding the pose for 10 to 20 seconds, then gradually increase the time to one minute.

Plank pose

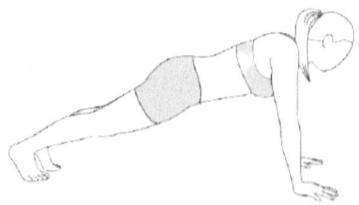

Spend ten to twenty minutes varying your plank pose.

1. Step your feet back with your heels lifted from the tabletop position.
2. With your body, form a straight line. Perhaps you'd like to examine your body in a mirror.
3. Contract your abdominal, arm, and leg muscles.
4. Maintain this position for at least one minute.

Chair pose

This pose is involved and very important for balance, which is necessary for weight maintenance and weight loss.

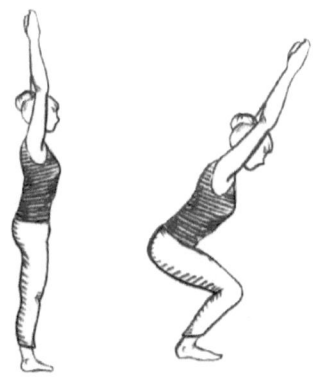

1. Keep your posture straight and your feet slightly apart.
2. Without bending your elbows, extend your

hands in front of you, palms facing downward.
3. Sit in a chair, bend your knees and push your pelvis down.
4. Raise your hand above your head, pointing your fingertips toward the ceilings.
5. In this position, lengthen your spine, look forward, and attempt to relax.
6. Take a moment to pause and inhale and exhale normally in the position.

Bow pose

The Bow pose engages your core, arms, and legs in a strong position.

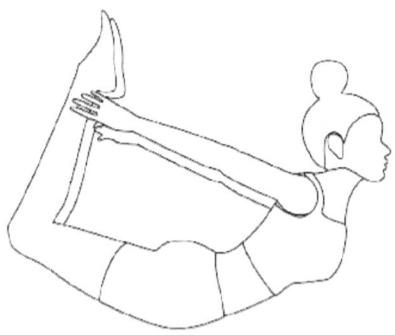

1. Lie on your stomach, hip-width apart, with your arms by your side.
2. Raise your knees and bring your heel towards your buttocks.
3. With both hands, grasp the ankles of both legs.
4. Inhale deeply and raise your chest and legs off the floor.
5. Maintain a straight face and pull your legs as much as possible. Your body should be taut, similar to a bow.
6. Take 4-5 deep breaths and then return to the starting position.

Cobra pose

Cobra pose is a fantastic pose to improve balance and flexibility.

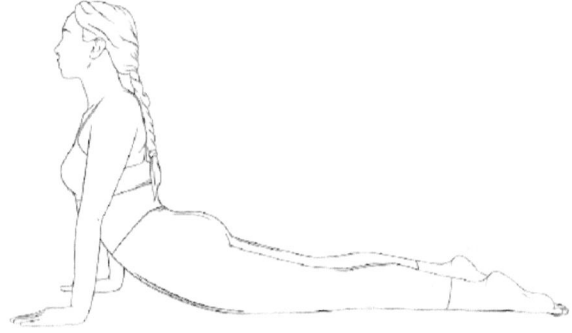

1. Lie on your stomach, feet together and arms stretched overhead.

2. Bring your legs together and place your forehead on the ground.
3. Tuck your hands beneath your shoulders (palms on the side of your chest), keeping your elbows close to your body.
4. Inhale and lift your upper body.
5. Exhale and hold for a few breaths in this pose.

If you want to use yoga to lose weight, you must commit yourself and practice. Make small, gradual changes and set modest goals to increase your likelihood of success.

As your practice and awareness develop, you may discover that you are naturally drawn to healthy foods and ways of life. While losing weight is not guaranteed, it is highly likely, and the benefits may extend well beyond weight loss to include increased energy, improved tempers, and well-being. You may find that you are "seeing the light" in yourself in ways you hadn't before.

Yoga is a powerful tool for healing your mind, body, and soul. It will assist you in clearing negative thought patterns, replacing them with positive ones, and breaking free from old habits that are no longer beneficial to you. It will help you overcome your fears and grow more confident in yourself.

SUPERFOODS TO AVOID FOR WEIGHT LOSS

There is a ton of knowledge available regarding the weight-loss benefits of specific foods. However, one group of foods has been ignored. Most of the nutrition literature ignores them because their benefits have been documented in a wide variety of ways.

This chapter will learn about the foods that are bad for you when consumed in excess and what one should consume to lose weight. This includes foods to avoid after a meal, before exercise, or as an additive in a meal. You will also learn why it matters to avoid these foods and what happens when you make these dietary mistakes.

This chapter is not intended to promote any particular diet. Instead, the goal is to help you make healthy choices about food for your body and mind. The focus is on using common sense to avoid certain foods because you recognize their toxic nature and know that they are not constructive to your health. When viewed in this light, it becomes clear why following some of these food recommendations may be difficult without support. This text supports and makes the process easier by detailing five superfoods for weight loss, why they should be avoided, what happens when you eat too many of them and their alternatives for healthy weight loss.

1. Caffeine

Caffeine is an alkaloid drug that stimulates the central nervous system. It is extracted from the leaves of coffee plants and other plants, including cocoa beans. It has been used for therapeutic purposes since the early 19th century, although its origin as a drug dates much further back. Its use as a medicinal agent declined in the 20th century with the discovery and commercialization of many safer drugs. Regardless, it is one of the most commonly prescribed medications in the US, with a wide range of potential health benefits and risks.

A psychoactive stimulant, caffeine is bad for you and shouldn't be part of your weight-loss plan. The small intestine rapidly absorbs it, its effects are felt nearly immediately. The effects of caffeine include:

1. Increased alertness and decreased fatigue
2. Improved reaction times and coordination
3. Enhanced mental clarity and focus
4. Stimulation of the sympathetic system and adrenal glands
5. Increased metabolic rate, heart rate, and blood pressure
6. Relaxation of smooth muscles in the bronchial tubes
7. Dilated blood vessels, allowing more oxygen to be delivered to the body's cells
8. Increased production of stomach acid, which stimulates digestion

Caffeine is also an effective diuretic. It will promote an increase in urination and a loss of water from your body. This can lead to dehydration. The net result is that a person will feel more awake and alert but less tired than if they had not consumed caffeine. This is why it is commonly taken during a workout or race.

It is important to note that caffeine can spell disaster for your diet by interfering with your body's balance of energy and nutrients. Your body becomes dependent on caffeine, so when you stop drinking it, you will experience withdrawal symptoms. These symptoms can include headache, fatigue, restlessness, disturbed sleep, muscle cramps and tremors, increased heart rate, and other problems. Most experts recommend avoiding caffeine if possible.

2. Alcohol

All forms of alcohol raise blood glucose levels more than other carbohydrates because alcohol breaks down into sugar in the liver before being absorbed by the small intestine. The risk of Type 2 diabetes, especially in women, maybe double for every glass of wine or regular beer consumed per day. Alcohol also has a high-calorie content, so that it will contribute to weight gain. Drinking less alcohol is an important part of any healthy diet.

When alcohol is consumed in excess, it can be toxic for the liver and other organs. This is especially true for people with a history of alcoholism and a compromised immune system. Cirrhosis of the liver and liver cancer can develop as a result of repeated liver damage.

Alcohol also inhibits the body's ability to recognize and utilize sodium and potassium, leading to abnormal heart rhythm and arrhythmias. As a result, alcohol consumption increases your risk of heart disease by four times that of people with no alcohol consumption.

Furthermore, heavy drinking can cause a condition known as alcoholic cardiomyopathy that can reduce heart function.

Alcohol is not healthy for any domain of life, and it should be avoided if at all possible during weight loss efforts.

3. Chocolate

It's crucial to keep in mind that chocolate is a food, not a drug. It is made from the seeds of the cocoa tree, which contains stimulants called amphetamines. These drugs are similar to caffeine and are part of the family of attention deficit disorder or hyperactivity drugs. The stimulants in chocolate impact your brain the same way as coffee, and other stimulants do, except that you feel it more slowly when you eat it instead of drinking coffee or another form of caffeine.

While chocolate may taste good, it has several side effects that make it bad for your diet:

- It usually prevents other foods from being digested properly because it causes stomach upset and constipation.
- It can contain up to 200 calories per ounce, so it is easy to consume more calories than you realize.

- It can cause insomnia, mood swings, and increase your risk of cardiovascular disease.
- It is extremely addicting, which is why people say they "love" chocolate and that they could "eat it forever."
- It can contribute to other conditions such as acne and zits if consumed in excess.
- It contains caffeine, which has already been discussed above.

Many people are unaware that they can indulge in chocolate as a treat, but they should reconsider. The quality of chocolate is also important; because it is made from the tree using only dark chocolate. Always read the ingredients and check the label to make sure you're eating only pure chocolate.

4. Sugar

Because of sugar, the obesity epidemic has become so prevalent in America. Sugar acts as a sweetener, so eating too much can cause weight gain and other unhealthy conditions.

While sugar is not the only contributor to obesity, it is one of the main factors because of how quickly it causes glucose levels to rise in your body.

Why does sugar make you fat? It quickly causes insulin levels to decrease after eating it, so you get hungry soon after eating it and then eat more food during your next meal than you normally would have. In addition, when you eat a lot of carbs, your body converts them into sugars for energy rather than using them for their intended purpose: building cells and tissue (protein) within your body.

While sugar is not healthy, it can be consumed in moderation as part of a low-carbohydrate diet, which is one of the most effective methods for losing and maintaining weight. Including some sugar in your diet does not mean you are eating a lot of carbs. For example, a slice of cake (which is not low in calories) does not mean you are eating a lot of carbs for the day. However, eating several cake slices will quickly add up total calories and carbs. In other words, moderation is key with sugar and all foods.

5. Fried Foods

While fried foods are high in fat and calories, they do not provide as much filling as you might believe. The consumption of fried foods has increased dramatically over the past century and is one reason why Americans have become so overweight.

The more saturated fat in your diet, the more likely you will get heart disease. This is because saturated fat raises cholesterol levels in your blood, clogs your arteries, and causes heart disease. Fried foods are usually high in trans fats or partially hydrogenated oils. Consuming too many trans fats can cause chronic inflammation throughout your body and increase the risk of developing diseases like cancer or diabetes.

Fried foods are hard to avoid completely because many thousands of them are sold in stores, but some of the best choices for your diet include nutrient-dense foods like vegetables, fruits, nuts, and seeds in their natural forms. Food manufacturers and restaurants often use high amounts of fat and calories in processed, fried foods rather than natural unhealthy fats like butter, avocados, or nuts.

Stick to natural, whole foods to lose weight, and avoid fried foods as much as possible.

SUPERFOODS FOR WEIGHT LOSS

Weight loss is a difficult goal to attain. Several factors come into play, including your body type, lifestyle, metabolic rate, and, most importantly, your level of physical activity and diet quality. Some foods are both nutritious and low in calories and thus can assist you in healthily achieving your weight loss goal. These foods are known as superfoods, and they're great for staying in shape. These superfoods not only provide your body with all of the necessary vitamins and minerals, but they also contain compounds that may aid in fat burning.

Here are ten superfoods that should be part of your weight-loss diet:

1. Apples

These delicious fruits have been shown to boost metabolism and suppress appetite, leading to weight loss. A daily apple could save you from more than just the doctor's office. It might even assist you in losing those extra pounds. Apples are high in antioxidants, dietary fiber, and essential vitamins and minerals. They're delicious to eat and extremely versatile. You can put them in breakfast cereals and salads for lunch and make healthy snacks and desserts with them in the evening.

2. Oatmeal

There is a reason that oatmeal is a weight-loss superfood. It is incredibly filling and contains both soluble and insoluble dietary fiber, which are two very important compounds for proper digestion, absorption, and elimination of food wastes in the body. Oatmeal also helps you feel full for a longer time after being consumed because of its complex carbohydrates and protein content. This can aid in weight loss because it keeps you from eating excess calories. It would help include oats as a part of a morning or afternoon snack. Studies have shown that eating these foods throughout the day may help you lose more weight than if you only eat them at one time.

3. Salmon

Salmon is another type of fish that has been recognized for its high weight-loss potential. Salmon is far healthier for you than red meat. It contains high amounts of omega 3 fatty acids, which have been found to reduce inflammation and lower cholesterol. Eating salmon daily can assist you in losing weight, especially around your waistline. The omega 3 fatty acids help reduce belly fat and keep your heart healthy. A diet rich in fish can also lead to higher metabolic rates. The protein found in this type of fish also helps slow carbohydrates in the body, so they are not converted into fat as quickly as otherwise. It is important to note that the fatty acids found in salmon can also replace trans fats, a type of fat found in processed foods. Trans fats are linked with several chronic diseases and have contributed to weight gain. Salmon is an excellent source of these fatty acids, abundant in cold-water fatty fish like salmon.

4. Green Tea

Green tea is rich in catechins, almost as powerful as caffeine. Catechins are what gives green tea its powerful antioxidant effects. They have been found to aid in weight loss by suppressing appetite and speeding up metabolism. According to one study, people who drink two or three cups of green tea each day lose a lot of weight than someone who does not drink any green tea. It is high in antioxidants, which protect the body from oxidative damage and aid fat metabolism. Green tea's antioxidant compounds also appear to be linked to its ability to reduce obesity and promote lean tissue mass. In addition, the caffeine found in green tea effectively decreases appetite.

5. Berries

Berries are one of the best superfoods for weight loss because they contain various vitamins and minerals essential to health, which can help reduce caloric intake while increasing metabolism. Additionally, they are high in fiber, which aids in digestion and weight loss by absorbing excess calories that would be stored as fat. Berries provide a fruit-like taste without calories, and sugar is usually present in other produce. There are numerous varieties available, so you're sure to find your favorite during your next grocery run.

6. Broccoli

Due to its high concentration of glucoraphanin, an anti-cancer compound, broccoli is one of the best superfoods for weight loss. It also contains indole-3-carbinol, which blocks the production of estrogen and prolactin and acts as a diuretic. Combining these two compounds aids in weight loss by decreasing both fat and water retention. This can help people who struggle with weight gain or maintain healthy body weight. Broccoli is a nutritious food and can be easily added to any meal or consumed as a snack. It could also potentially replace certain types of bread or pasta that you may be eating regularly.

7. Flaxseed

Flaxseed is another type of superfood high in Omega-3 fatty acid. It also contains lignans, which have been shown to help curb appetite and improve weight loss by preventing the breakdown of body fat and reducing its absorption, which is a common cause of weight gain. This can also be achieved by consuming flaxseed in supplements or on its own, making it an excellent food choice for weight loss. It is usually added to oatmeal and other baked goods to increase dietary fiber and protein content.

8. Olive Oil

Olive oil is another superfood high in polyphenols, which has been shown to aid weight loss by suppressing appetite. It has also been linked with decreased body fat, a common cause of weight gain. Olive oil is an excellent source of monounsaturated fatty acids, omega-3 polyphenols, and phenolic compounds. These healthy oils are good for heart health and reduce bad cholesterol levels. They also help improve blood circulation, leading to better heart health.

9. Grapefruit

Grapefruit contains resveratrol, which has been linked with burning calories and lowering the risk of heart disease. Grapefruit contains resveratrol, which has been linked with burning calories and lowering the risk of heart disease. It also contains naringin, a compound that has been shown to promote fat loss by impacting the body's metabolic rate. A study found that people who drank grapefruit juice for two weeks lost more weight than those who did not take it every day. Resveratrol has also been linked with improved blood sugar levels, leading to weight loss. Grapefruit is also high in pectin, which lowers LDL cholesterol and promotes healthy blood sugar levels.

10. Sweet Potatoes

Sweet potatoes are a nutrient-dense food containing complex carbohydrates and dietary fiber to aid in digestion. They are sweet and are high in beta-carotene (a form of vitamin A), lutein, zinc, and several other vitamins and minerals. These healthy oils reduce the amount of fat absorbed by the body and help decrease cholesterol levels that contribute to heart disease. They also contain a good source of dietary fiber, which reduces insulin levels, favoring weight loss.

11. Strawberries

A great superfood for weight loss, but in some cases, the best way to lose weight is to maintain a healthy diet, especially if you have been struggling for quite a long time. Strawberries are packed with vitamins and minerals, antioxidants, and phenolic compounds that enhance the health of skin and cells. According to many studies in rats, strawberries can even delay the onset of diseases such as cancer or Alzheimer's disease by encouraging cell protection mechanisms in the body. In addition, strawberries can help prevent type 2 diabetes by lowering blood sugar levels in patients with this disease. Strawberries are also high in fiber, which aids in the absorption of vitamins and minerals.

12. Garlic

Garlic is another superfood that can help you lose weight by maintaining an overall healthy diet. Garlic contains a high concentration of antioxidants, which help prevent free radicals from damaging cell tissue and causing aging or disease. Also, garlic assists with regulating blood sugar levels in the body and aids in weight loss by decreasing appetite and improving metabolism. According to one study, taken together, these two qualities combine to help people successfully maintain their weight loss after 8 weeks of ingesting garlic in a supplement form. Garlic is also high in fiber, which can aid digestion and can help the body absorb some of the nutrients it contains.

13. Ginger

Unprocessed ginger is a good source of antioxidants and dietary fiber, which contributes to normalizing stomach acidity and increasing metabolism. Ginger also helps with weight loss by decreasing appetite and reducing cravings for unhealthy foods. It also has anti-inflammatory properties that can help reduce swelling in the subcutaneous tissue. The natural components in ginger could help make it a superfood that aids in weight loss, but adding it to your diet may take some getting used to if you are not used to having lots of spices. Additionally, it has anti-inflammatory properties that aid in weight loss by decreasing blood fat and inflammatory markers. These qualities make it a highly effective food for coping with weight gain or maintaining healthy body weight. Ginger may also benefit patients who have heavy menstrual cycles due to its ability to combat inflammation and pain while balancing hormones. Ginger is high in fiber, which can aid digestion and provide you with energy.

14. Spinach

This is another superfood that benefits the body's health in many ways, including aiding in weight loss. High in fiber and packed with calcium, iron, vitamins A, C, K, protein, and other antioxidants, help prevent heart disease and cancer. Additionally, it contains beta-carotene (a form of vitamin A), which aids in the maintenance of a healthy immune system. Additionally, it contains beta-carotene (a form of vitamin A), which aids in the maintenance of a healthy immune system. Spinach is good for your heart to reduce cholesterol levels and improve cardiovascular function. This food can also help you lose weight by increasing your calorie expenditure during exercise.

15. Cauliflower

Not only is cauliflower high in fiber and antioxidants, it also contains a high concentration of vitamin C, which has been connected to weight loss and can help improve skin elasticity and immunity. Furthermore, this vegetable is rich in lutein and zeaxanthin, which protect against eye diseases. It also contains a glycoprotein called stevia that helps boost fat burning process in the body.

Superfoods are a fantastic source of nutrition and can easily aid in weight loss. Some superfoods have also been linked with lowering cholesterol levels, which prevents heart disease. Using these foods, you can maintain a healthy body weight and lose weight simultaneously.

THINGS TO AVOID WHILE TRYING TO LOSE WEIGHT

Weight loss can be difficult for some people. Even if you believe you are leading a healthy lifestyle, you may be falling short of the results you desire. You may be following outdated or incorrect advice. This may prevent you from noticing the changes you desire in your body or from losing the pounds you desire.

HERE ARE 15 COMMON WEIGHT-LOSS BLUNDERS THAT PEOPLE MAKE

1. Concentrating solely on the scale

When you look at the scale every day, it becomes a measure of your success instead of a true indicator of how you are doing. If your weight fluctuates, it cannot be easy to trust that your efforts are working.

Despite leading a healthy lifestyle, it's common to feel like you're not losing weight quickly enough.

It is critical to remember that the number on the scale represents only one measure of weight loss. Several factors influence weight, including fluid fluctuations and the amount of food left in your system.

Your weight may fluctuate by 2 to 4 pounds over a few days, depending on how much food and liquid you consume.

This happens because you'll gain weight when you drink a lot of liquid — say, 8 to 10 cups of water a day. Drinking that much fluid decreases how much space remains in your digestive tract. As a result, the amount of food sitting in your gastrointestinal tract will decrease as well.

With that information in mind, try not to be discouraged if the numbers on the scale don't align with your expectations. Instead, stay focused on how you look and feel.

2. Obsessing over "bad" foods

When you decide what foods are off-limits, it's tempting to overindulge in them just because they're forbidden fruits. Are you skipping the sugar bowl because you're determined to lose weight and then eating a bowl of ice cream?

The more specific you are about which foods you're cutting out, the more food-obsessed you might become. Are you attempting to cut back on your fast food consumption? If so, it's probably not a good idea to frequent fast-food restaurants. Those places will make your longing for their fat and sugar-filled treats worse.

If you are serious about eating healthier, it's important to avoid the foods that are most likely to sabotage your goal. Instead, focus on your diet and the nutrients you'll get from healthy foods.

3. Excessive or insufficient calorie intake

You can't lose weight if you're not eating enough calories. Although two women may be the same age, height, and weight, a woman who weighs 130 pounds has different caloric needs than one who weighs 170 pounds.

Your daily calorie requirement is determined by your gender, size, and lifestyle. For example, if you are very active and play sports, you need more calories than someone who is sedentary or doesn't participate in sports. But even if you eat fewer calories than you should, your weight-loss efforts will stall or fail. You'll want to calculate the number of calories you're consuming and make adjustments based on the information. You can use a tracking app to help keep an eye on your calorie intake and expenditure. Say, for instance, that you're eating 1,500 calories a day but not losing weight. In this scenario, it's time to reduce that number by 500 calories for a week or two.

If you consume less than 1,000 calories per day but continue to gain weight, you should gradually increase your daily calorie intake by approximately 250 calories per week. This will ensure that you're not undernourished and gain muscle.

In one study, adults were asked to run on a treadmill, estimate how many calories they burned, and then a meal with the same number of calories. According to the study, participants significantly underestimated and overestimated calories in exercise and food.

You may be eating foods like nuts and fish that are healthy but high in calories. The importance of eating moderate portion sizes cannot be overstated.

On the other hand, severely limiting your calorie intake can backfire. Very low-calorie diets have been shown to cause muscle loss and significantly slow metabolism in studies.

4. Exercising too little or too much

We hear about the importance of exercising so much that we often do too much exercise. The truth is, you don't have to work out more than 45 minutes a day to burn calories and lose weight.

An excessively high-intensity workout could also lead to muscle loss.

It's time to change your routine if you're used to spending hours at the gym every week and are looking for effective ways to lose weight. You don't have to spend hours at the gym each week. You don't have to train for marathons. As long as you're following a healthy diet, you'll see results.

If you don't exercise at all while calorie-restricting, you're more likely to lose muscle mass and have a lower metabolic rate.

If you don't exercise at all while calorie-restricting, you're more likely to lose muscle mass and have a lower metabolic rate.

Exercising, on the other hand, maybe beneficial:

1. Retain as much lean mass as possible
2. Enhance fat loss
3. Keep your metabolism from slackening

4. Reduce your risk of heart disease and diabetes
5. Improve your mood and brain function

It's important to exercise in moderation, doing a few cardio sessions each week. Do some endurance exercises instead of going to the gym if you don't have time to go. Endurance activities can help you burn fat while maintaining muscle mass.

Overexercising can be problematic. Excessive exercise, according to studies, is unsustainable in the long run for most people and can lead to stress. Furthermore, it may harm endocrine hormones, which help regulate body functions like metabolism, sleep, and mood.

5. Focusing on appearance over health

Many people who decide to lose weight focus on their appearance rather than their health. Luckily, there are effective ways to help you lose weight without subjecting yourself to unsafe diet plans or dangerous plastic surgery procedures.

When you're focusing solely on your appearance, it's tempting to resort to extreme weight loss methods like crash diets or even anorexia. These methods may help you shed pounds quickly initially, but they take a toll on your body in the long run. They can also make you feel emotionally unstable and leave you vulnerable to eating disorders like bulimia or binge-eating disorder.

Instead, focusing on the health benefits of eating a balanced diet and maintaining a healthy weight would be beneficial.

Several of the health benefits you'll enjoy if you follow this advice include the following:

1. Improve your energy levels and moods
2. Lower blood pressure and triglycerides (blood fats)
3. Reduce the risk of heart disease, diabetes, and certain cancers (colorectal, breast, prostate)
4. Lower cholesterol levels in your bloodstream

6. Lifting no weights

When you focus on weight loss rather than strength training, you're missing out on one of the best ways to lose fat.

Weight training helps you build muscle mass, which helps burn fat and maintain a healthy metabolism. You should aim for 30 minutes of strength-training sessions each week, but any amount of time spent exercising is better than none.

The impact of weight training is particularly beneficial in your first few weeks of weight-loss dieting. During this period, your body is at its maximum caloric burn-- meaning that it weighs the least. It's critical to focus on your muscles rather than just cutting calories from your diet, especially in the early stages of weight loss.

As you lose weight, you'll need to make some adjustments to your exercise routine.

For instance, if you're on a low-carb diet and start losing muscle mass, it's time to reduce the intensity of your workouts. Keep up the endurance training and moderate weight training sessions. If you're losing muscle mass despite a small calorie deficit, it's time to up your daily calorie intake by 250 to 500 calories.

If you're lifting the right amount of weights, your muscle mass will improve. As a result, you'll notice changes in your body composition: your waistline will shrink, and your belly fat will decrease. If you have belly fat, you may even notice it decrease on its own, as many people do.

7. Avoiding protein and cooking food at higher temperatures

Some people believe that eating a high-protein diet is how to lose weight. When you consume a lot of protein, you might think that your body won't absorb the calories, but this isn't true. The body will absorb all of the calories it needs regardless of carbohydrates or fat. If a person consumes an extreme amount of protein about fat, they may experience water retention.

You'll need to consume a lot of protein if you want to lose weight. Some people recommend getting an extra five grams of protein per day (or following other diets with similar proportions) from food.

Additionally, if you're trying to lose weight, you should avoid frying foods and instead prepare them at lower temperatures. Frying food at high temperatures can change the coating on the food, making it harder for your body to break down and digest. Instead, try grilling or steaming food instead.

8. Not planning meals

Many people assume that when they're following a weight loss diet, it won't change their lifestyle much. They get fast food when they're out running errands and prepare quick meals when they realize that their daily schedule is too busy for food prep.

If you're looking for effective ways to lose weight, though, your diet will have a huge impact on your overall health. If you pass up the opportunity to plan your meals each week and don't leave time to prepare them, you'll be eating unhealthy foods like preservative-laden frozen dinners or junk food out of convenience.

Instead, try this simple approach to planning meals: Buy or make a week's worth of food. Get recipes online or at cookbooks that you like, and then plan your meals each week. This approach is more economical because you won't have wasted food during the week and no empty packages to throw away the following day.

If your family eats at home a lot, you can set up a weekly "dinner night" where you prepare one meal at the same time every night. For example, dinner might be leftovers from the following day's lunch. It also helps if you freeze prepared foods in portions that will last several days.

9. Eating a lot at night

Many people eat more at night than during the day because their schedule is busier or their digestive system slows down. If you're trying to lose weight, you'll want to avoid this habit. It's important to stop eating well before bedtime, especially if you're trying to lose weight quickly.

When you eat a large meal late at night, your body will struggle to process it the next day. Rather than burning calories and fat in your sleep, your body will store excess calories as fat. This can leave you with added pounds that are hard to shed.

Instead of eating at night, try eating small, healthy meals during the day. Don't worry about overeating--make sure you don't eat every three hours or skip meals. If you do this, you'll increase the calories that you burn overnight and ultimately lose weight more quickly.

10. Not eating enough fiber

If you aren't eating enough fiber, you might inadvertently sabotage your weight loss efforts.

When fiber is present, it helps you feel full and eat fewer calories. For instance, whole grain bread and cereals are full of fiber, as are lentils and beans. However, many people don't eat enough fiber because they don't want to feel full or have been told that they should eat less of the food during weight-loss diets. Although fiber doesn't have a main role in helping you lose weight, it does have several benefits that will help you feel better and breathe more easily.

The best way to get the most benefit from your dietary fiber intake is to consume whole foods--fruits and vegetables--before cooking or processing them into foods like bread or muffins where their fiber content has been lost. If you don't bother eating whole food, be sure to eat a lot of fiber.

If you're trying to lose weight, it's smart to ensure that you're getting enough dietary fiber. If you eat a high-fiber diet, your digestive system will benefit from increased waste removal and regularity, which can help keep the weight that you've lost steadily.

If your digestive system is functioning well, your body will regulate its fat content more effectively, which will burn fewer calories and use less energy overall. Additionally, some studies have shown that people who consumed more fiber had lower BMIs than those who didn't consume as much fiber.

11. Overestimate the number of calories burned during exercise

If you are trying to lose weight and burn more calories, you may think you can eat more if you burn a lot. But the research on calorie expenditure during exercise concludes that the number of calories burned during exercise is highly dependent on your body weight, the intensity of work, and time.

Furthermore, it is not that easy to overestimate the number of calories burned during exercise. When people worked out moderately, they tended to underestimate their calorie expenditure by as much as 70%.

When it comes to losing weight smartly, be sure not to fall into this trap. Make sure to burn more calories than you consume, and understand that your body weight will dictate how many calories you burn during exercise. Otherwise, you'll be wasting time and money on less-effective weight-loss strategies.

Additionally, suppose you're going to burn more calories than what you consume. In that case, it's best to get leaner and not try all kinds of alternative methods--which could result in counterproductive results.

It's not a big surprise--the scientists said that the human body is designed to conserve energy during times of starvation. However, if you want to make sure you're healthily losing weight, keep moving and eating healthy.

12. Not getting enough sleep

It is critical to get enough sleep for your physical and mental health. It helps regulate your hormone levels, boost your immune system, and provide your body with much-needed rest.

So, if you're trying to lose weight, it's especially important to make sure that you're getting plenty of rest and avoiding sleepless nights. Sleep deprivation has been shown to increase the hormone ghrelin, which stimulates hunger, and cortisol, which is known to promote fat production.

If you constantly don't get enough sleep or suffer from insomnia, do what you can to improve your sleep. Limit your caffeine intake and avoid eating late at night. Keep in mind that the best time to go to bed is around 10 pm--so try not to eat dinner before this time.

You'll be able to cope with stress without gaining weight if you get enough sleep each night. Likewise, you'll get more energy throughout the day because your blood will flow better--which means that your metabolism will work faster.

If you don't sleep enough, you'll find it difficult to manage stress and your cravings, which means you'll be more likely to give in to food cravings. This will not only make it harder for you to lose weight, but it will also cause your body to store excess fat.

It's critical to remember that the amount of sleep you require will vary depending on your circumstances, such as working long hours or having a large family to care for. Start with about 7 hours a night, and work your way up from there as needed. If this sounds too much for you, consider consulting your doctor first.

13. Unrealistic expectations

It's easy to overestimate your dieting ability when you don't understand losing weight. For instance, if you don't know that eating fruit and vegetables is an important part of losing weight, it's easy to be disappointed in yourself--even though the number of calories you're eating doesn't seem low enough to be effective.

It's also important for dieters not to expect too much from themselves at first--especially in terms of weight loss. While everyone is different, studies show that most people will only lose 1-5 pounds per month when starting a diet--and this rate can slow down as time goes on.

If you're trying to lose weight, don't be discouraged if the scale doesn't budge at first--it will take time. However, it's important to do what you can to speed up the process by following a healthy diet and incorporating daily exercise. Also, remember that while exercising may not burn as many calories as some forms of exercise, it still helps you burn more calories overall--so try to incorporate it in your daily routine.

The weight-loss process will go much faster if you keep moving and doing small things consistently each day. Get off the couch, take a walk around the park or neighborhood every 30 minutes (or even 10 minutes), and make sure to get moving with your work-outs too.

If you're following healthy eating habits and working out because you think it will help you lose more weight, understand that your exercise routine is also an important part of your overall weight loss program--so make sure to follow it regularly. In other words, no matter how much or how little weight you want to lose, if you want the best results, practice what works best for you.

14. Not understanding which foods to eat and which not to

This mistake is often made by people new to dieting who assume that eating all the foods on the list will help them lose weight--which is not true.

So how do you know which foods to eat and which to avoid? Once you understand that it's not about what you're eating, but rather about how much of it you're eating, it becomes a lot easier. You don't have to be a picky eater--focus on making healthy food choices most of the time. This includes increasing fruit and vegetable consumption, whole grain consumption, lean protein consumption (such as chicken or fish), and water consumption.

Boil it down to this: The best foods for losing weight include fruits, vegetables, whole grains, lean proteins, and water. For instance, if you're cutting back on your caloric intake to lose weight, try increasing how much of these foods you eat instead. Similarly, if you're trying to control your appetite (or eat healthier), once again--increase the amount of these foods that you consume each day.

This isn't to say you shouldn't eat other foods; rather, eating healthier foods is the most effective way to lose weight. If you're trying to lose weight, don't just follow a diet plan that's based on fruits and vegetables; read the nutrition label first. This will help you understand the number of calories contained in the food, which can help you gain a better idea of the number of calories in each portion.

One way to see if you're eating enough or too many calories is to track your daily food intake for two weeks and see your average calorie intake. If you're eating too many calories, adjust your diet accordingly and try to burn more calories through exercise.

Even if you eat all the right foods--and eat them in moderation (i.e., not as a meal)--you can still gain weight by being lazy when it comes to exercise. This is because muscle weighs more than fat, so you might see a big difference in your weight even though your body becomes more toned and healthy.

You can't lose weight effectively by relying solely on dieting or exercise; you'll need both.

15. Not tracking your progress

This mistake is made by people who are hopeful that they will lose enough weight to fit into their old clothes--without knowing how much weight they might have to lose.

Many people find it easier to make dieting changes if they measure their progress in some way--which is why measuring your body fat percentage can be a great way for you to track your progress and see if your goals are within reach. Another advantage of measuring body fat percentage is that it allows you to set more realistic goals. For instance, you should track how much time you spend exercising, what foods you eat, and how much weight you lose each week.

This practice will let you identify patterns in your eating habits and workout routine, which can help you make adjustments that lead to better results.

If it's not working for you, do something different--but how will you know that it worked? It all comes down to understanding which parts of your diet and exercise program are working (or not) and making adjustments accordingly.

To know if you're doing something right, you need to track your progress. This includes keeping a food journal, tracking your workouts, measuring your weight and body every week, writing down how you feel at the end of each day and every week--and reading up on healthy eating and exercising habits. It sounds time-consuming, but it's worth it in the long run.

Letting your guard down for even a week can undo all the good you've done. So make sure to stay focused--especially during week 1, when it's the most important for weight loss. If you slip up just one time, don't be discouraged--get back to following your diet and exercise plan when possible.

To achieve maximum results, plan to spend 20-30 minutes each day on your exercise routine--whether that's a morning workout, a workout at lunchtime, or a night workout.

And remember: it is not about the scale--it's about what you see in the mirror. Also, don't forget to monitor your progress by looking at your weight over time and comparing it with photos of yourself before you start dieting.

While there are a variety of approaches to losing weight, the most important thing is to avoid setting yourself up for failure from the start. This means not looking for a quick-fix solution, starting with realistic goals and then focusing on losing weight for the long run.

If your diet and exercise program is not working for you, do something different. Remember that small adjustments over time will get you to your goal much faster than dramatic diet changes every month or so. Concentrate on eating healthy foods, exercising on a regular basis, and keeping track of your progress. That's all there is to it.

LOSING WEIGHT TOO FAST

Although you want to avoid setting yourself up for failure, it's also important to be realistic. It's natural to lose weight too fast. After all, if you're trying a diet that does not include food portions or making drastic changes in your daily routine, you might expect that you'll start seeing results very fast.

But remember that losing weight is not about making drastic changes or diet fads and schemes--it's about making healthy lifestyle changes over time.

On the other hand, if you start dieting too quickly and don't give your body enough time to adjust to your new lifestyle habits, you could experience side effects and possibly even crash. This is because you'll burn fewer calories than what you're eating, so eventually, your body will turn into a fat-storage machine.

When it comes to weight loss, the adage "slow and steady wins the race" applies: don't go overboard, or you'll end up in a dieting disaster. Overall, it's best to focus on losing 1-2 pounds per week to prevent crashes and health issues. With that said, you can still lose weight faster by changing your workout routine and eating a bit less each day but be careful not to go overboard.

While you can lose weight too fast, there's also such as losing weight too slowly. Keep track of your progress or meet with a weight loss expert once or twice a month to see how you're doing to avoid this happening to you.

While there are numerous methods for losing weight, the best approach is to begin by eating well and exercising regularly. As was mentioned earlier, you can try different diets and exercise routines to see what combination works best for you, but don't go overboard. Smaller changes over time will get you where you want to be faster than drastic diet changes every month or so.

10

CALORIES IN FOOD AND CALORIE

Sometimes, it's hard to know how many calories you're eating or how many calories you need to lose weight. Most nutrition facts labels don't give you the full story. They provide the number of grams of fat, carbohydrate, and protein in a food item.

This might work for people who want an idea of what they're eating, but this isn't enough information for people who want to lose weight. For example, if a food item has 100 calories and 10 grams of fat per serving but only has 2 grams of protein, it's obvious that it isn't great for weight loss.

A few online calories and nutrition counters provide further information, such as protein, carbohydrate, and fat in a food item. While they take some time to figure out how to use these tools and keep track of your meal intake, they're worth it if you want to lose weight.

A calorie is an energy unit. Calories in nutrition refer to the energy people get from food and drink and the energy they expend during physical activity.

CALORIE INFORMATION

1. Calories are necessary for human survival.
2. Calories are required by the body to rebuild and maintain itself.
3. Everyone requires different amounts of energy throughout the day, depending on their age, gender, size, and level of activity.
4. The body stores energy to use later.
5. The body uses energy at the rate of 1 kcal per hour.
6. The human body expends more energy than it consumes daily, allowing for maintenance and regeneration during sleep.
7. Calories in food can be burned or stored.
8. Calories are measured in many units, including kilocalories (kcal), which measure the energy content of food and drink, and calories per gram, which is used to measure the energy content of human tissue.

9. The number of calories you get from your diet represents only 20 percent of your daily caloric intake; 40 percent comes from other sources, such as drugs, tea, and alcohol.

Most people associate calories with food and drink, but calories can be found in anything that contains energy.

Calories are divided into two categories:

1. Small calorie

Your body uses these to help maintain its balance of fluids, minerals, and vitamins.

2. Large calories

These provide energy during physical activity.

Researchers believe that the human body has a basic metabolic rate of 100 kcal per day, varying according to age and gender.

At body temperature (37°C), the small calorie is roughly equal to the number of molecules required to add one gram.

The number of calories in food is measured in kilocalories (kcal) or calories per gram.

> 1,000 calories are equal to 1 kcal.

"Large calorie" and "small calorie" are frequently used interchangeably. This is deceptive. Kilocalories are the unit of measurement for calorie content on food labels. A 250-calorie chocolate bar has 250,000 calories in it. A small calorie is the unit of measurement for energy expenditure.

The food label shows how many kilocalories or kcal the food contains. The caloric equivalent and the number of small calories are not provided on the label.

Daily requirement

The quantity of energy or calories required to keep our bodies functioning and healthy varies depending on our age, gender, height, weight, and level of physical activity.

- Women need between 1,600 kcal and 2,000 kcal a day, depending on their activity level.
- Men need between 2,000 kcal and 3,000 kcal a day, depending on their activity level.
- Male athletes require more calories than women because they have larger muscles that use more energy to move during exercise.
- An overweight person requires more calories than an average-weight person.

The Harris-Benedict equation is a popular method for calculating calorie needs. This helps predict how many calories a person requires depending on their gender, activity level, height, and weight. Although it might underestimate calorie needs for active people, it can accurately estimate the caloric requirement of sedentary people.

The equations are as follows:

Male: 65 + (13.7 x weight in kg) + (5 x height in cm) - (6.8 x age in years) = daily kilocalories required to maintain current weight.

Female: 655 + (9.6 x weight in kg) + (4.7 x height in cm) - (4.8 x age in years) = daily kilocalories required to maintain current weight.

If you want to lose weight, it's recommended that you take advice from your doctor before starting a diet.

The calorie intake for a healthy person is about 2,000 kcal per day when not actively engaged in exercise. This number will increase when someone exercises and decreases based on the number of calories burned.

Calories and health

To survive, the human body requires calories. The body's cells would die without energy, the heart and lungs would stop beating, and the organs would not carry out the basic processes required for survival. However, individuals vary—the average adult human needs between 2,000 and 3,000 kcal per day.

The Recommended Dietary Allowance (RDA) is the recommended amount of nutrients daily to meet our nutrient requirements. In 1976, the Institute of Medicine's Food and Nutrition Board developed the RDA. The values are a healthy man weighing 70 kg (154 lb) and an average-sized woman weighing 57 kg (126 lb). Just as important as the calories themselves is the substance from which they are obtained.

The calorific values of three major food components are listed below:

1. Carbohydrates have a caloric value of 4 kcal per gram.
2. Each gram of protein contains 4 calories.
3. Each gram of fat contains 9 calories.

As an example, here's how one cup of large eggs, weighing 243 g, would provide calories to a person:

23.11 g fat
207.99 kcal = 23.11 g x 9 kcal
30.52 g protein
122.08 kcal = 30.52 x 4 kcal
1.75 g carbohydrate
7 kcal = 1.75 x 4 kcal

347 calories are contained in 243 grams of raw egg. Fat provides 208 kcal, protein provides 122 kcal, and carbohydrates provide 7 kcal.

Empty calories

Contrary to popular belief, empty calories do not contain any nutrients to improve the health of the human body. Calories that provide energy but have little nutritional value are empty calories. Dietary fiber, amino acids, antioxidants, dietary minerals, and vitamins are all lacking in foods high in empty calories.

Solid fats

Although they are found naturally in many foods, they are frequently added during industrial food processing and preparation. Solid fat is something like butter, and it is found in foods like cookies, doughnuts, pastries, biscuits, frozen desserts, prepared vegetables like fast foods, and snack foods.

Sugars

Refined sugars contain simple sugars that are used for energy. For example, glucose and fructose are types of sugar. There's also sucrose. Refined sugars and sugar substitutes (high fructose corn syrup) can be empty calories because there is no fiber present to slow the absorption rate of the sugars into the bloodstream.

Empty calories are commonly found in any product that provides 5 or more grams of sugar or one serving's worth of refined grains per day. Since it is difficult to eat just one serving of most foods containing empty calories, it is easier to consume these calories in snack food or processed food. Added sugars and solid fats enhance the flavor of foods and beverages. They do, however, add a lot of calories and are a major contributor to obesity.

Sources of empty calories

The following foods and beverages contain empty calories:

Added sugars and solid fats

- Donuts
- Pastries
- Cookies
- Ice cream
- Cake
- Candy
- Soda pop
- Corn chips
- Popcorn
- Doughnuts
- Pastries, sweet
- Other baked goods and desserts
- Fruit drinks (high sugar content)

Solid fats

- Butter, margarine
- Shortening
- Canola oil (vegetable oil)
- All types of cooking oils
- Olive oil

- Palm oil
- Lard and other animal fats (beef, mutton, pork, etc.)
- Margarine and other spreads (usually hydrogenated)
- Milk fat (butter)
- Hydrogenated oils
- Cream, sour cream (usually from milk fat)
- Cheese, including cottage cheese and ricotta cheese
- Beef
- Pork and ham
- Butter, margarine
- All types of vegetable oils (corn oil, soybean oil, safflower oil, sunflower oil, etc.)
- All types of cooking oils (olive oil included)
- Animal fats (beef and other animal fats)

Added sugars

- Fruit drinks
- Non-diet soft drinks
- Sodas

Processed foods containing refined grains (e.g., white bread, white rice, etc.) are usually high in empty calories. It's worth noting that some foods that appear to be healthy may actually be high in empty calories. For example, a candy bar may only have 200 kcal, but it still contains empty calories because vitamins and minerals do not contain sugars. Large amounts of refined grains can cause heart disease and diabetes over time.

There are ways to find products that are lower in solid fat and empty sugars. For example, instead of a standard hot dog or a fatty cheese, a person could opt for low-fat options for both.

Empty calories can be avoided or drastically reduced by incorporating fresh, healthy food and drink into one's diet.

Carbohydrates are a major source of energy. Despite that, they have been the subject of many negative studies. This may be because carbohydrates tend to be high in calories.

People who eat a high-carbohydrate, low-fat diet are more likely to gain weight, especially around their stomachs, according to research. Carbohydrate intake can stimulate the secretion of insulin and cortisol, two hormones that affect fat storage. There is some evidence that certain carbohydrate types (carbs with a high glycemic index) can raise blood sugar levels, increasing hunger and leading to overeating.

Calories may appear to be linked only to weight gain and obesity, but they are necessary for good health. Only when consumed in excess of the recommended amount, can they be harmful to one's health.

When calculating calories, you should consider not only your diet but also your level of physical activity. Regular, high-intensity exercise can help offset a high-calorie intake.

Many exercise machines can track the number of calories burned. Some require manual input from the user regarding the duration and intensity of their workout to calculate calories burned or BMI. These machines can be found in gyms and health clubs and include treadmills, elliptical trainers, stationary bicycles, rowing machines, stair-steppers, and cross-country ski simulators.

CALORIE DEFICIT

A calorie deficit is simply a negative calorie intake. To make up the deficit, one must expend more calories than they take in. The two ways that calories can be ingested and expended are through food and exercise.

Calories expended during weight loss and maintenance are a combination of physical activity, such as walking, and caloric restriction. If a person chooses to consume fewer calories than they expend in energy, they will lose weight.

Calories consumed more than calorie expenditure will lead to weight gain or weight retention. A person will not lose weight if they consume more calories than they expend. For healthy weight loss, most doctors and nutritionists recommend combining both changes.

Exercise more

Exercise burns calories and, in turn, helps you create a calorie deficit. Exercise does not have to be intense or complicated. Exercise burns calories and, in turn, helps you create a calorie deficit. Exercise does not have to be intense or complicated. Any activity, from gardening to biking to walking, is beneficial. Even a short walk in the morning can help increase metabolism and burn calories throughout the day.

You don't have to complete everything at once. Shorter 10-minute bursts can be done throughout the day.

Before beginning a rigorous exercise program, consult your doctor, especially if you are overweight or have other health issues.

Remember that even if you don't lose weight, regular exercise can help you stay healthy. It prevents your body from gaining weight. It also aids weight maintenance if you have lost weight.

Reduce calories by eating less

Eat fewer fats and sugars, and avoid processed foods made with white flour, added sugars, and unhealthy fats.

How to eat fewer calories

1. Eat more vegetables

It would be beneficial if you consumed more vegetables than fruits and a variety of them. You must consume fewer calories from carbohydrates such as fruits and grains in order to lose weight. At the same time, you need to increase your intake of vegetables and legumes. You can do this by making sure at least half of your plate is covered with fresh or frozen vegetables at every meal. You can also choose healthier options like lean meats in place of carbohydrates.

Some examples of Vegetables and how many calories it has:

- Cabbage = 25 calories per cup shredded
- Broccoli =30 calories per cup chopped
- Cauliflower = 25 calories per cup chopped
- Arugula = 35 calories per cup raw salad
- Watercress = 30 calories per cup raw salad
- Kale = 20 calories in ½ cup raw salad, blanched or sautéed.
- Spinach = 17 calories per cup raw salad
- Brussels sprouts = 30 calories per cup shredded or chopped
- Leeks = 35 calories per cup gourmet stir-fry or braised.

- Lettuce = 15 calories per cup shredded.
- Cucumbers = 20 calories per cup chopped.
- Green beans = 20 calories per cup cooked.
- Bok choy = 40 calories for 1 cup stir-fried or braised, 25 for 1 cup raw.
- Tofu = 50-100g raw tofu contains 33-80 calories depending on the firmness and size of the pieces and whether it is fried or not.
- Winter Squash = 30 calories for 1 cup cooked and mashed.
- Green Peppers = 50 calories per cup chopped and cooked.
- Peppers = 20 calories per cup raw
- Celery = 20 calories per cup chopped cooked or raw
- Onions = 40 calories per cup chopped, raw or sautéed
- Tomatoes = 25 calories for 1 large tomato (raw) 100g cherry tomatoes contain 18-25 Calories depending on the cherry size. One medium tomato contains 32 calories
- Potatoes (with skin) = 160-180 cal for 100 g boiled, baked, or mashed potatoes and about 200-220 cal for the same amount of French fries.
- Lima beans = 50 calories per cup raw
- Beans (black) = 100 cal per cup

- Beans (kidney) = 100 cal per cup Cooked in boiling water or instant powder. Fava bean has 50 calories per cup, and green beans have 140 calories per cup cooked.

You can include cabbage, cauliflower, arugula, and kale in your diet. Just be sure to prepare them properly. Cooking or boiling these would consume a lot of their nutrients and boost their calorie count greatly, from 20 calories for a half-cup of raw salad to 70 calories for a half cup of cooked salad.

2. Eat more fruits

Fruits are a critical component of a balanced, healthy diet. They contain vitamins and minerals, fibers, and carbohydrates in an easily digestible form. There is no need to cut out fruits from your diet if you are trying to lose weight; however, you should eat fruit more sparingly. One serving is approximately the size of one apple or one banana per day. If you want to lose weight, reduce this amount to 1/2 of the serving size every day. If you do so moderately, there is no reason why you would not meet your calorie targets for the day.

Examples of Fruits and how many calories it has:

- 1 medium banana = 50 calories
- 1 medium apple = 83 calories

- 1 cup de-stemmed strawberries = 32 calories (½ cup)
- 2 medium oranges = 90 calories each (¾ cup)
- 3 large plums = 88 calories each (¾ cup)
- 4 cups grapes (1 pound) = 72 calories each (½ cup)
- 2 cups honeydew = 110 calories each (1 cup)
- 1 medium pear = 95 calories
- 1 cup raspberries = 80 calories (1 cup)
- 1½ cups cherries = 85 calories (1 cup)
- 1 medium mango, peeled + pit removed = 100 calories
- 1 medium pear, unpeeled + pit removed = 90 calories
- 1 large pineapple, peeled + cut into chunks = 149 calories (½ cup)
- 3 medium nectarines, peeled + pit removed = 125 calories (1 cup)
- 2 cups blackberries (1 pound) = 110 calories each (½ cup)
- 5 medium plums = 120 calories each (¾ cup)
- 100g blueberries = 45-70 cal per 100 g depending on the color of the berries.
- 100g strawberries=44-62 cal per 100 g depending on the color of the berries. (½ cup)
- 1 medium apple or 1 banana= 50 calories.
- 100g raspberries = 60 calories. (½ cup)

- 1 medium orange= 62 calories.
- 1 medium peach= 66 calories
- 2 medium kiwi= 58 calories
- 100g mango= 55-65 cal per 100 g depending on the color of the mango. (½ cup)
- 1 cup strawberries = 50-65 cal per 100 g depending on the color of the berries
- 200g pineapple = 80-115 cal per 100 g depending on the color of the pineapple. (½ cup)
- 3 medium apricots, fresh or dried= 70-85 cal per 100 g depending on the color of the fruit. (¾ cup)

3. Eat more lean Protein

The majority of people consume enough protein on a daily basis, but not all of it is natural and nutritious. A large portion of the protein we consume comes from meat, such as red meat, chicken or turkey, and dairy products. While red meat has many proteins and is good because it can increase muscle mass, it contains fats which is an essential part of our body's metabolism system and cause many problems like heartburn, high cholesterol level, etc. You should consult your doctor before reducing your consumption of red meat. While chicken and turkey have many essential proteins, they are mostly water.

As a result, finding alternative protein sources to aid weight loss is critical. The most common protein sources in our diet are beans, peas, and lentils. Aside from being rich in proteins, these vegetables are also low in the glycemic index and are high in fiber which aids heart function, maintains a healthy digestive system, and lowers cholesterol levels and blood pressure. Also, eating lots of leafy greens will provide you with natural proteins since they contain chlorophylls and other essential nutrients for cell repair and tissue growth.

You can also eat tofu and nuts. Because tofu is made from soybeans and is high in protein but low in calories, it should be combined with other ingredients to balance the protein and carbohydrate proportions. Nuts have a lot of calories (150 to 200 for one ounce) but are not high in Protein. You are supposed to eat them sparingly since they are rich in fats.

Alternative sources of protein include:

- Navy beans - 6 g Protein per 100 g
- Soybeans - 4 g Protein per 100 g
- Honeydew melon - 4 g Protein per 100 g
- Tofu - 2.5 g Protein per 100g
- Kidney beans - 1.5 g Protein per 100 g
- Lentils - 1.4 g Protein per 100 g

- Oats - 1.3 g Protein per 100g
- Broccoli - 1.2 g Protein per 100 g
- Quinoa - 1.1 g Protein per 100g
- Chia seeds - 2.6g Protein per 100g
- Hemp seeds - 2.5g Protein per 100g
- Leafy greens, collards - 2.3 g Protein per 100g
- Spinach - 2.1 g Protein per 100 g
- Kale - 1.9 g Protein per 100g
- Wheat bread - 1.4 g Protein per 100g
- Tofu - 3.6 g Carbohydrates per 100g (½ cup)
- Almonds - 40.5 g Protein per 100 g
- Coconut - 72.95 g Protein per 100 g (1 cup)
- Walnuts - 18.7 g Protein per 100g (½ oz)

The required Protein for a calorie deficit is 0.8g per lb of body weight.

To reach the protein requirements for fat loss, you must eat more whole foods and less processed foods. It is better to eat more portion sizes of lower calorie count than a few portion sizes of the high-calorie count. Crash diets are not recommended because they are not long-term sustainable and will only cause you to gain weight once you resume your normal eating habits. It will also aid your goals if you eat mostly lean meats and keep refined carbohydrates out of the picture while increasing your fiber intake.

4. Change your snack.

In between meals, many people reach for a snack or two. Snacking is acceptable, but select lower-calorie options. When hunger strikes, the key is to have some healthy snacks on hand. In between meals, many people reach for a snack or two. Snacking is acceptable, but select lower-calorie options. When hunger strikes, the key is to have some healthy snacks on hand. Nuts and dried fruits are great sources of protein, fiber, and healthy fats. These snacks can also satisfy your craving for something sweet. It is a good alternative to choose almonds or fruits instead of your regular chips.

A handful of nuts contains more protein than a candy bar, and let's face it, and nuts are far more satisfying than candy.

5. Remove one calorie-dense treat from your diet

Each day, try to eliminate one high-calorie food item. If you are a morning coffee drinker, cut back to one cup. If you have a favorite dessert, eat it only once or twice a week instead of every day. If you're a connoisseur of chocolate, swap out your regular chocolate for a dark variety instead. This technique will help keep daily calorie counts in check and ensure that you eat more whole foods than processed ones.

6. Do not consume your calories by drinking

When you take in your calories through drink, you increase your risk of becoming overweight and obese. The calories from drinks are often forgotten when counting calories. Juices and carbonated sodas may be high in calories but lack essential nutrients. When it comes to consuming fluids, water is the best option. It also has no calories, which is perfect for weight loss.

7. Add more fiber to your diet

The most important factor is to eat at least 30 grams of fiber per day.Fiber will help you feel full, decrease cravings, help stabilize blood sugar levels and enhance digestion. Aim for 40-50 grams of fiber a day to lose weight and 100 grams per day if you want to manage your condition to keep it off. Load up on the fruits and vegetables high in fiber like celery, sweet potatoes, and apples, then eat the ones you don't care for but still need the nutrients from like blackberries, blueberries, raspberries, and strawberries. Don't forget to include the whole fruit and not juice. The fiber is usually destroyed in the juicing process, so you are not getting the juice's proper amount of fiber. Adding a fiber supplement along with eating plenty of fruits and vegetables will help you reach your daily goal faster.

Losing weight is never easy, but if you follow the steps above, it can be a more rewarding experience than exhausting. It takes hard work, dedication, and a change in lifestyle for weight loss to be effective in the long run. Hopefully, the above information will help you see that slimming down is possible when you start with small changes in your day-to-day life.

THE DAILY PERCENTAGE VALUE (DV%)

The Percent Daily Value (percent DV) for each nutrient in a serving of food is the percentage of the Daily Value for that nutrient. The Daily Values are nutrient amounts to consume or not exceed daily to reduce the risk of chronic disease. The DV measures the percent of a nutrient in a typical serving. Protein, fat, carbohydrate, and water provide the energy and nutrients needed to perform daily functions. The DV is calculated using a 2,000-calorie diet that meets or exceeds the RDA for each nutrient (RDI).

The DV is obtained by dividing the percent for each nutrient in food by the RDI for that nutrient. The RDI is based on both total daily intake and normal physiological needs nutritionally. For example, a food that contains 100% DV for calcium and less than 10% DV for iron is low in calcium and high in iron. Similarly, a food that contains 100% DV for sodium but less than

10% DV of vitamin C is high in sodium but low or lacking in vitamin C.

The percent DV for a nutrient is found by dividing the amount of the nutrient in that food by the Daily Value for that nutrient. For example, in a serving of chicken noodle soup, 100% DV for sodium is 50% DV for sodium/calories and 100% DV for calories, but 100% DV of one (The Daily Value Total) and 50% DV of another (The Daily Value Percent) equal 50%. Thus, the percent DV for sodium would be 50%.

Each %DV value on this page has been calculated using "The Daily Values." The Daily Values are based on a 2,000 calorie diet, and "The Daily Value has been adjusted so that 2,000 calories a day is equal to 1,600 calories of fat, and other calorie amounts are the same, except for protein which is 8% lower.

Follow this easy math to determine how much of each nutrient should be consumed per day to minimize the risk of chronic disease and promote healthy aging.

The daily values have been adjusted so that a 2,000 calorie diet is equivalent to 1,600 calories of fat and other calorie amounts are the same except for protein which is 8% lower.

12

GETTING TO AND MAINTAINING YOUR IDEAL WEIGHT

You'll feel more energized and like you're living the life of your dreams as you exercise more and keep your diet in check. You'll also notice that you're losing weight, which is a great bonus.

However, it's important to achieve your health goals concerning your ideal weight and lifestyle. It would help if you always strived to be healthier than you are now. You shouldn't expect to lose weight overnight or in a short period.

To succeed in the long run, you need to set realistic goals and plans.

Here are some key points on losing weight, staying healthy, and maintaining your ideal weight:

11 THINGS TO KNOW BEFORE YOU START LOSING WEIGHT

1. Even if you exercise regularly, it may take several weeks or months before you see results.
2. When you exercise regularly, your metabolism slows down. You need to increase your calories and decrease your activity level if you want to achieve a positive weight loss.
3. When you first wake up, drink water and start slow before eating breakfast or lunch. For meals to digest, the food needs to pass through the stomach for some time. Before eating, eat a snack about three hours after your last meal at night. This will give you enough time before breakfast or lunch to digest the meal properly
4. If you aim to lose weight, drink at least eight glasses of water each day. Drinking this amount of water will help your body function better.
5. Don't pass up breakfast; it's the most important meal of the day. It jump-starts your metabolism and gives you plenty of energy to face the day.
6. When eating a large meal, try chewing more and spending little time between meals. It will

help you eat less and is a healthier way to consume food instead of swallowing too much at once quickly.
7. Keep your bedroom cool to sleep better and stay healthy, especially if you want to lose weight overnight or over a short period without exercise
8. If you're trying to lose weight, eat fruit for dessert instead of cake or candy.
9. If you're trying to lose weight but don't like to exercise, do a little at a time and work up from there. When exercising, drink plenty of water so that your body will stay hydrated and healthy.
10. To lose weight quickly, cut down on eating carbs and eat more protein instead.
11. Make your juices by putting fruits into the blender and blending until thoroughly mixed, then drink it after an hour or so before each meal.

Enjoy your life and don't worry about details too much. Once you reach your goal weight, maintaining it is easy. Your body will adjust to the weight number it is at, so work on yourself within this range, and your calorie intake will naturally decrease once you've reached that goal weight.

Never stop researching ways to lose weight, whether through dieting or exercise. Remember to take breaks if you feel exhausted, and remember that treating yourself also means always eating healthily and exercising. Get a good night's rest, and make sure you take your vitamins each day. A healthy diet and regular exercise are the way to go if you want to lose weight and stay healthy.

RECIPES FOR CALORIE DEFICIT

Green Bean and Mushroom Soup (250 calories each serving)

Ingredients

- 1 medium chopped onion (60 calories)
- 2 cloves minced garlic (10 calories)
- 3 cups chopped green beans, fresh or frozen (30 calories)
- 1 tsp olive oil (extra virgin) (40 calories)
- cup chopped mushrooms, fresh or frozen (20 calories)
- 1 bay leaf (0.N cal)
- 1/2 cup green peas (50 calories)
- 2 tablespoons flour (45 cal) or whole wheat flour (55 calories per cup)

- 2 cups water or vegetable stock (0 calories)
- salt and pepper to taste.

Preparation

1. Heat oil in a large saucepan or Dutch oven over medium heat. Add onion and garlic and sauté for 5 minutes.
2. Add green beans, mushrooms, salt, and pepper to taste, tossing in the pot until the beans are hot.
3. Remove all but 1 cup of the cooked green beans into a food processor or blender and blend until pureed, often stopping to scrape the downsides of the bowl with a clean spoon as you go along.
4. Add blended green beans back into the saucepan and stir in flour until well mixed.
5. Add the vegetable stock, bay leaf, peas, and water to the pan and heat through, stirring frequently.

Calories 250 (per serving)
Total Fat 3 g (Saturated Fat 0 g,
Polyunsaturated Fat 0 g, Monounsaturated Fat 0 g)
Protein 10 g
Carbohydrate 44g (Fiber 8 g, Sugars 11g)

Kale, Tomato, And Cheese Frittata (350 calories each serving)

Ingredients:

- 1 tablespoon extra virgin olive oil (40 calories)
- ½ cup chopped onion (35 cal)
- 1 ½ cups chopped kale leaves (40 calories) if you like cheese, add 1 tablespoon shredded cheese of your choice.
- ½ cup sliced cherry tomatoes (80 cal), halved or quartered if large; seeds removed (30 calories). If you want olive oil instead, use 1 tablespoon of the olive oil and a tablespoon of your favorite store-bought pesto. Anything else can be substituted.
- 1 medium egg (70 calories)
- ½ cup skimmed milk (50 calories)
- 2 cups shredded mozzarella cheese (200 calories). Shredded mozzarella is preferable, as it is faster to melt than fresh cheese. If you don't have shredded cheese, you can use a brick of mozzarella cheese (8 oz) and a package of extra-sharp cheddar or gouda to get the same effect.
- 1 teaspoon dried oregano (0 calories)
- 1/2 teaspoon dried basil (0 calories)
- Salt & pepper to taste.

Preparation

1. Heat oil in a 10-inch ovenproof nonstick skillet over medium heat; add onions and sauté, occasionally stirring, for 5 minutes or until tender.
2. Add kale and cook until wilted, stirring occasionally; sprinkle with tomatoes and stir to combine.
3. Whisk together egg, milk, ½ cup of shredded cheese, and herbs until smooth; pour into skillet.
4. Season scallop with salt and pepper.
5. Cook, stirring occasionally, until the egg sets on the bottom of the skillet, about 5 minutes.
6. Place the pan in the oven for 8 minutes, or until golden on top.
7. Remove from oven and sprinkle with remaining cheese; cover loosely with foil and let stand for 2 minutes before slicing.

Calories per serving: 350 (per serving)
Total Fat 15 g (Saturated Fat 4.17 g
Trans Fat 0 g
Cholesterol 145 mg (42%)
Sodium 410 mg (18%)
Total Carbs 26 g (Fiber 1.7 g)

Dietary Fiber 2.3 g (8%)
Sugars 12.2 g
Protein 29.8g

Roasted Vegetable Salad (260 calories per serving)

Ingredients:

- 1 cup baby spinach (140 calories)
- ½ cup roasted red bell pepper slices (50 calories)
- 2 tablespoons balsamic vinegar (20 calories)
- 1 teaspoon extra virgin olive oil (14 calories)
- ¼ teaspoon dried basil (0 calories)
- 1/8 teaspoon salt (0.7 g).
- ¼ teaspoon white or black pepper flakes or freshly ground black pepper to taste.

Preparation:

1. Combine all ingredients and let sit for 5 minutes.
2. Serve over a bed of mixed greens and enjoy.
3. Add ½ cup of chicken or turkey breast to make this a complete meal and add 40 calories per serving.

Calories 260 per serving

Total Fat 8 g (Saturated Fat 0.32 g
Trans Fat 0.00 g
Cholesterol 0 mg (0%)
Sodium 215 mg (9%)
Total Carbs 22 g (Fiber 2.1g)
Dietary Fiber 2.1g (8%)
Sugars 3.2 g
Protein 8.0 g

Broccoli, Chickpea, and Quinoa Salad (200 calories each serving)

Ingredients:

For the dressing:

- 1 tablespoon extra virgin olive oil (100 calories)
- ¼ cup fresh lemon juice (50 calories). If you prefer white wine vinegar, it has 4 g less of the same carbohydrates.
- ¼ teaspoon salt, or to taste.

For the salad:

- ½ cup chickpeas (100 calories)
- 1 medium head broccoli florets (60 calories), stems, and leaves separated using a sharp knife.

- 3 cups arugula or collard greens (45 calories)
- 4 medium mushrooms, sliced thin (10 calories). Any mushroom can be substituted with equal amounts of other mushrooms, such as portobellos, butternuts, or oysters.
- ½ cup almond slices (100 calories).
- ½ cup quinoa flakes (100 calories).
- 1 ½ teaspoon Dijon mustard (5 calories) (optional)

Preparation:

1. Combine dressing ingredients in a large bowl.
2. Cook quinoa according to package instructions and set aside to cool.
3. Blanch broccoli in boiling water for 2 minutes, or until crisp-tender, drain, and set aside to cool
4. Combine all ingredients and toss to combine.
5. Set aside to allow flavors to melt while preparing the mushrooms.
6. Slice mushrooms in half and place them in a medium-size skillet, drizzle with 2 tablespoons of the dressing, cover vegetables, and cook for about 5 minutes on medium heat or until tender, stirring occasionally.
7. Plate your salad on individual plates, top with

quinoa, chickpeas, broccoli florets, and arugula greens, then drizzle the remaining dressing over and enjoy.

Calories per serving: 200
Total Fat 13 g (Saturated Fat 1.5 g)
Trans Fat 0 g
Cholesterol 0 mg
Sodium 340 mg (15% DV)
Total Carbohydrates 8 g (Fiber 2.5 g)
Dietary Fiber 2.5 g (10%)
Sugars 3 g
Protein 8g

Stuffed Red Peppers with Sweet Potato (190 kcal per serving)

Ingredients:

- 1 medium sweet potato (134 calories)
- ¼ cup pesto sauce (50 calories)
- ½ cup cooked quinoa (100 calories)
- 2 tablespoons lemon juice, divided (10 calories). White wine vinegar can be substituted, but it will add 4 g more carbohydrates.
- ½ teaspoon salt, plus more to taste.
- 4 bell peppers (160 calories)

Preparation:

1. Prepare the pesto by whisking all ingredients in a small bowl or blender until smooth.
2. Steam the sweet potato for about 20 minutes, or until tender, then set it aside to cool; cut into small chunks, then combine with diced onion, grated cheddar cheese, and pesto. Mix thoroughly and refrigerate for 30 minutes to allow flavors to meld.
3. Combine quinoa, lemon juice, and salt in a mixing bowl and set aside to cool.
4. Preheat the oven to 425°F (300°C).
5. Remove the tops of the bell peppers, remove all of the seeds, and cook the peppers in boiling water for about 20 minutes, or until tender.
6. Once they are tender, drain and replace them in the pan to keep warm while preparing the quinoa mixture.
7. Fill each pepper with a heaping spoon of sweet potato mixture, top with quinoa mixture, and bake for 5 minutes or until quinoa is thoroughly heated through and starting to brown on top (if desired).
8. Remove from the oven and immediately serve with a large salad of your choice on the side.
9. Add ½ cup of chicken or turkey breast to make

this complete meal and add 40 calories per serving.

Calories per serving: 190
Total Fat 10 g (Saturated fat 0.93 g)
Trans fat 0 g
Cholesterol 0 mg (0%)
Sodium 265 mg (11%)
Total Carbohydrates 13.7 g (Fiber 2.2 g)
Dietary Fiber 2.2g (10%)
Sugars 5.9g
Protein 5.8 g

The Sweet Potato and Quinoa Salad (200 calories per serving)

Ingredients:

- 4 cups sweet potato, shredded (400 calories)
- ½ cup cooked quinoa (100 calories)
- 4 oz. feta cheese, crumbled (200 calories).
- ½ cup scallions, sliced thin (10 Calories)

For the dressing:

- 1 teaspoon balsamic vinegar (20 calories)
- 1/8 teaspoon garlic powder or ½ teaspoon granulated garlic (0.5 g). You can also substitute

1/8 teaspoon of minced garlic if desired. Leave out if you're not a fan of garlic flavor.

Preparation:

1. Cook the sweet potatoes and quinoa according to package instructions and let cool.
2. Toss all ingredients together until thoroughly combined in a large bowl or on individual plates, then drizzle with dressing and serve

Calories per serving: 200
Total Fat 10 g (Saturated Fat 3.2 g)
Cholesterol 8 mg (3%)
Sodium 395 mg (17%)
Total Carbohydrates 22 g (Fiber 4.3g)
Dietary Fiber 4.3g (18%)
Sugars 3.5 g
Protein 6.5 g

Thai-Style Peanut Noodles (140 calories each serving)

Ingredients:

- ½ cup cooked quinoa (100 calories)
- 1 / 4 cup peanuts, chopped (70 calories).
- 1 / 4 teaspoon ground cayenne pepper. More or

less can be added to make it as spicy as you like.
- 4 oz. Tofu, diced (60 calories). Add 30 calories per serving for a complete meal by adding 2 eggs with 20 g of lean protein each.
- 2 cups grape tomatoes, halved (20 calories). It can be replaced with other tomato varieties, including cherry tomatoes if desired.
- 1 tablespoon lime juice (5 calories)

For the dressing:

- 2 tablespoons lime juice (10 calories) or white wine vinegar (if you wish to reduce the carbs).

Preparation

1. Steam the grape tomatoes, tofu, and peanuts for about 5 minutes, or until heated through.
2. In a large mixing bowl or on individual plates, combine all of the ingredients until well combined, then drizzle with dressing and serve immediately.

Calories per serving: 140
Total Fat 0.11 g (Saturated Fat 0.09 g)
Trans fat 0.1 g

Cholesterol 0 mg (0%)
Sodium 340 mg (15%)
Total Carbohydrates 16 g (Fiber 3.5 g)
Dietary Fiber 3.5 g (14% DV)
Sugars 4.5 g
Protein 8g (11% DV)

Quinoa Salad with Kale, Quinoa, and Feta, and Pomegranate Seeds (180 calories per serving)

Ingredients:

- 1 cup cooked quinoa (140 calories)
- 1 tablespoon water (4 calories). You can add more or less to make it less or more soupy and add 10 calories per serving.
- ¼ cup feta cheese, crumbled (80 calories).
- ½ cup fresh pomegranate seeds, or dried quinoa or cranberries (40 calories)
- ¼ cup raw spinach, chopped (1 g) (can be substituted with other greens like kale or collards)

For the dressing:

- 1 tablespoon balsamic vinegar (20 calories).

Preparation:

1. Combine ¾ cup of quinoa with 1/4 cup water in a saucepan; cover and cook over medium heat for 15 minutes, occasionally stirring until water has been absorbed.
2. Meanwhile, cook the kale for 5–7 minutes. (Set aside to cool.)
3. Combine crumbled feta cheese, pomegranate seeds, cooked quinoa, and spinach in a salad bowl; season with additional balsamic vinegar if desired. Toss until combined and add dressing to taste.

Calories per Serving: 180
Total Fat 1 g
Trans Fat 0 g (0% DV)
Cholesterol 0 mg (0%)
Sodium 500 mg (20%)
Total Carbohydrate 25 g (Fiber 6.7 g) (19% DV)
Dietary Fiber 6.7 g (32% DV)
Sugars 5 g
Protein 9 g (18% DV)

Quinoa with Carrot and Raisin Mix (205 calories per serving)

Ingredients:

- 1 cup cooked quinoa (160 calories). You can also substitute quinoa flakes or cooked lentils if desired.
- ½ cup carrot, finely grated (30 calories). You can substitute this with other vegetables like broccoli or zucchini, but you'll need to add extra water. For example, ¾ cup of broccoli florets have 25 calories, so you'll need an additional ¼ cup of water to cook it.
- ½ teaspoon ground cinnamon (3 calories)
- ½ teaspoon ground ginger (3 calories)
- ¼ teaspoon nutmeg (1 calorie)
- Several raisins, chopped (50 calories).

For the dressing:

- 1 tablespoon low-fat mayonnaise (80 calories). 1 tablespoon of whole fat mayo will add 60 calories per serving. If you wish to reduce the carbohydrates, you can substitute with 6 teaspoons of extra virgin olive oil and ¼ teaspoon mustard. This would add 90 extra calories per serving.

Preparation:

1. Combine the cooked quinoa, shredded carrot, raisins (or any other dried fruit you like), and spices in a medium-sized bowl.
2. Mix until well combined.
3. Drizzle with dressing and serve immediately.

Calories per Serving: 205
Total Fat 8 g
Saturated Fat 1 g
Trans Fat 0 g
Cholesterol 0 mg (0%)
Sodium 160 mg (7%)
Sugars 6 g
Protein 7 g

Kale salad with grilled chicken (205 calories per serving)

Ingredients:

- 2 cups kale, stemmed, chopped (chopped kale is a better option because it retains more nutrients.)
- 1 cup cooked quinoa (160 calories)
- ½ cup grilled chicken breast, shredded (95 calories).

- 1/3 cup fresh cilantro, chopped (20 calories). You can substitute with parsley if desired.
- ½ teaspoon lemon juice (0 calories)
- Optional seasoning: 1 teaspoon Worcestershire sauce or dry mustard powder and ½ teaspoon liquid smoke. The Worcestershire sauce will add about 5 calories per ½-tablespoon serving, while the liquid smoke will add about 7 calories per ½-tablespoon serving.

Directions:

1. Heat a medium-sized skillet to medium heat and add 1 teaspoon of extra virgin olive oil. Stir in kale with the seasonings for about 2 minutes. Remove the pan from heat, then atop each serving plate, add chopped kale, shredded chicken breast, and cilantro. Drizzle lemon juice over each plate and garnish with additional cilantro (optional).
2. Serve warm or cold! You can prepare this dish in bulk by mixing all ingredients in one large bowl, dividing it into 6 servings, and storing it in a covered container in the refrigerator for up to one week.

Calories per serving: 205

Total Fat 8 g
Saturated Fat 1.3 g (6% DV)
Trans Fat 0 g (0% DV)
Cholesterol 70 mg (23%)
Sodium 370 mg (16%)
Total Carbohydrate 21 g (Dietary Fiber 4.7 g (22% DV)
Sugars 0.1 g
Protein 17 g

Shrimp fajitas (200 calories per serving)

Ingredients:

- 1 cup cooked quinoa (140 calories). You can substitute quinoa flakes or cooked lentils if desired.
- 1 ½ pounds peeled and deveined shrimp (100 calories).
- ½ teaspoon ground cumin (3 calories).
- ¼ teaspoon paprika (2 calories).
- ¼ teaspoon chili powder (1 calorie).
- ¼ teaspoon garlic powder (2 calories).

For the salsa:

- ½ cup red pepper, chopped (40 calories)
- ½ cup tomato, chopped (20 calories)
- ¼ cup yellow onion, chopped (10 calories)

- ¼ cup fresh cilantro, chopped (20 calories).
- Several fresh lime wedges (about 2 per serving) (optional).

Directions

1. In a bowl, combine shrimp and season with cumin and paprika. Heat a medium-sized skillet to medium heat and add 1 teaspoon of extra virgin olive oil to the pan; stir in shrimp until well combined and cooked through, about 2 minutes per side. Remove the pan from heat, then atop each serving plate, add shrimp and chopped vegetables. Add garlic powder and season with salt to taste.
2. Top with optional salsa and lime wedges on the side.
3. Serve warm or cold! You can prepare this dish in bulk by mixing all ingredients in one large bowl, dividing it into 6 servings, and storing it in a covered container in the refrigerator for up to one week.

Calories per serving: 200
Total Fat 6 g
Saturated Fat 0.5 g (3% DV)
Cholesterol 90 mg (30%)

Sodium 450 mg (19%)
Total Carbohydrate 12 g (Dietary Fiber 1.8 g (7% DV)
Sugars 2 g
Protein 24 g

Crockpot Quinoa with veggies (235 calories per serving)

Ingredients:

- 1 cup quinoa (160 calories) (then you can add soy sauce and tofu if desired!)
- 2 teaspoons extra virgin olive oil (40 calories). You can substitute with non-hydrogenated vegetable oil or canola oil if desired.
- 1 medium onion, diced (50 calories). You can substitute with shallots if desired, but they will add about 10 extra calories per ¼-cup serving.
- 2 small carrots, peeled and diced into small pieces (32 calories). If desired, you can substitute with parsnips or celery root, but it will add about 40 extra calories per ¼-cup serving.
- 1 cup frozen peas (30 calories). If desired, you can substitute with any other vegetable, but it will add about 70 extra calories per ¼-cup serving.
- 1 teaspoon dried rosemary (3 calories)

- 1 teaspoon chili powder (0 calories)
- ½ teaspoon dried parsley or basil, finely chopped (0 calories). You can substitute with cilantro if you wish, but it will add 30 calories per ¼-tablespoon serving.
- If desired, you can add 1 tablespoon of soy sauce for about 10 extra calories and 1-ounce tofu for about 55 extra calories.

Directions:

1. Heat the quinoa in a small saucepan with 1 teaspoon extra virgin olive oil for about 10 minutes, or until fully cooked. Then toss with all vegetables except for the peas—Cook for about 30 minutes on low heat. Serve warm or cold.
2. Prepare this dish in bulk by mixing everything in a large bowl, dividing it into 4 servings, and storing it in a covered container in the refrigerator for one week.

Calories per serving: 235
Total Fat 5 g (Saturated Fat 0 g) (Trans Fat 0 g)
Cholesterol 0 mg (0%) (excludes salt added during cooking)

Sodium 405 mg (18%) (excludes salt added during cooking)
Total Carbohydrate 35g (Fiber 4g, Sugars 5g)
Dietary Fiber 4g
Sugars 5g
Protein 7g
(24% DV if using shrimp with bones and skin.)

Eggplant Dip (290 calories per serving)

Ingredients:

- 1 tablespoon extra virgin olive oil (40 calories)
- ½ cup chopped onion (35 cal)
- ½ cup chopped celery (40 cal), or 1 medium stalk of celery, chopped.
- 2 cloves minced garlic (10 calories)
- 1 tablespoon flour (15 cal) or whole wheat flour (45 calories per cup)
- 1 28-ounce can crushed tomatoes or 2 cups fresh tomatoes, crushed by hand in a blender or food processor.
- 1 teaspoon dried basil (0 calories)
- ½ teaspoon dried oregano (0 calories)
- 1/8 teaspoon salt (0.7 g).
- ¼ teaspoon white or black pepper flakes or freshly ground black pepper to taste.

Preparation:

1. Heat oil in a medium saucepan for a few minutes over medium heat. Add onion and celery, and sauté, occasionally stirring, for 5 minutes or until slightly softened.
2. Add garlic and sauté for 30 seconds.
3. Add flour and cook, stirring, for 2 minutes.
4. Bring tomato sauce, basil, oregano, salt, and pepper flakes to a boil in a saucepan.
5. Add mixture to the pan and stir until thickened, about 10 minutes.
6. Remove from heat and allow to cool slightly before using.
7. Serve with crackers, cheese sticks such as string cheese or cheese cubes, or use as a dip for vegetables or toasted bread slices.

Calories per serving: 290 (per serving)
Total Fat 12 g (Saturated Fat 2.33 g
Trans Fat 0 g
Cholesterol 0 mg (0%)
Sodium 880 mg (37%)
Total Carbs 32 g (Fiber 5.5g)
Dietary Fiber 5.5g (22%)
Sugars 7.8 g
Protein 6

CONCLUSION

There are a handful of things you should do that will help you lose weight and feel good. The key here is to figure out what is important to your life, what going up a few notches on the scale means for you, and then take small steps in the right direction. There are many different ways to do it, and all of them take time, work, and commitment. The most critical thing a reader can do is to develop and adhere to a plan that fits their lifestyle. The key to success is consistency. A large percentage of people who try to lose weight fail because they do not stick to their diet and exercise routine. They think it will be easy, but it rarely is.

Learning the essentials in dieting and doing them regularly will help you the most. Start with what you already know if you want to lose weight quickly. Start easy and build up slowly over time. Be patient and never give up. You will succeed if you put your whole heart and soul into it. The benefits of losing weight are magnificent. You will look and feel fabulous, and it will help you live a healthier life for years to come.

The best diet is a diet that you can stick to. Don't make drastic changes too soon, or you will get discouraged and give up. People who start a new diet usually gain the weight back once they stop. It might take months to lose weight, but it takes only a couple of weeks to gain it back. The key is consistency in a carefully crafted plan that works for your lifestyle.

Losing weight isn't something that happens overnight, nor can it be done on the spur of the moment. Some people think that it will be simple and quick, but this is mostly not true. If you want to lose weight, you must make small lifestyle changes and stick to them over time. It will take a while before the changes are felt, but the weight loss begins. Losing weight isn't a sprint; it is a marathon.

The best thing is finding a good diet plan that works for you and then staying with it. If the weight doesn't come off quickly enough, don't get discouraged – this is normal. Slowly but surely, it will come off eventually. Once you have reached your goal weight and maintained it for a few weeks, then go back and tweak your diet plan so you can keep losing more fat and not gain it back again. There are natural ways to tone down your body and keep it that way without harming your health.

You must allow your body to change over time. If you go on a crash diet, you will only lose the water weight that your body holds onto. It is meant to hold onto it to survive. When your body feels stressed, it holds on tighter to this water. It is an instinct that has been around for thousands of years. Losing weight can take some time, but once the weight loss starts, you will slowly notice changes in your body every day, and eventually, it will become a new way of life for you.

Begin losing weight immediately after making the decision to do so. Exercising will assist you in losing weight and maintaining it. Exercising is a fantastic way to shed those extra pounds. Exercising will give you the energy you need and make your body more toned and fit. If you want to start exercising, go ahead and do it, as long as it doesn't cost a fortune or make you feel guilty about exercising.

Consistency is the key to real change in life, whether good or bad. Doing yoga helps with stress and weight loss. It can also calm your body and mind in a way that nothing else can. Make sure that you take the time for a daily yoga session to lose weight, feel good, and have more energy.

To lose weight, begin by making small changes to your daily habits. Instead of taking the elevator, take the stairs, or go for a walk during lunch or right after work. Exercise will help keep off extra pounds and tone up your body, which is one of the keys to losing weight. Your diet may not be perfect yet, but these tips will help you eat better today than yesterday and tomorrow than today until you get to your goal weight.

Bring a nutritious lunch from home to work. It will save you money and calories, and you won't have to worry about what unhealthy options are available at the office. You will feel better by eating less fast food and focusing better when you don't have that distraction in your mind because of how hungry you are. Drink at least eight cups of water a day, but not all in one sitting. Drink it throughout the day, as well. If you are thirsty, drink it with your meal or between when you eat so that you won't feel hungry again soon after. Your body needs clean and clear water to function properly. You will have fewer cravings if you stay hydrated, but more importantly, staying hydrated keeps your skin healthy and plump. There are many things to avoid when you are trying to lose weight.

One way to lose weight is to eat less often so that even when you are full, you can still eat less. Calorie Deficit is one way of eating less and not breaking your diet. It means that you don't eat whenever you feel hungry, but only when full. This can be accomplished by eating smaller portions and keeping track of the foods you consume. If you are always hungry, maybe it is time to try a small change to your diet to help you lose weight.

Cut down on the amount of sugar in your drinks and snacks. Alcohol, soda, candy, and other sugary foods all encourage weight gain, which everyone needs to watch out for if they want to lose weight successfully. If you want to lose weight, try to eliminate all sugary foods as much as possible.

Reduce your weekly grocery bill by shopping around for lower-priced items. Look for the sales, coupons, and deals that can save you money at your favorite stores. Find out when the stores have their grocery sales and stock up on the items you need to make your meals healthy and tasty.

Don't just eat one serving of vegetables per day, but eat a wide variety of vegetables throughout the day. Once cooked, most vegetables do not increase in volume much at all, so they can be eaten with little danger of gorging yourself or leaving any behind before you reach your destination. It would help meet your daily nutrient needs to lose weight and keep it off. Make sure that you consume your vegetables, whether cooked or raw.

When preparing meals ahead of time, think about what will be done with the leftovers. For large amounts of leftovers, double the recipe and freeze half for later use. That way, you have a healthy portion ready for reheating later on in meal form.

Setting up an exercise routine can be one of the hardest parts of losing weight for some people. It can be hard to keep motivated if you start running and don't know how or where to go. Try finding a place where you enjoy doing the activity, such as a local park. If it is cold outside when you work out, start small. Start by walking on a track and seeing how far you can get before your legs give out on you. Gradually increase the distance. You'll be running for miles before you know it.

Cooking for yourself will give you much more control over the type of food you ingest. This enables you to prepare your meals in a calorie-conscious manner. You can also eliminate any food you are not fond of by cooking for yourself. If you learn new recipes, it will be easier to make your meals and not worry about what the restaurant offers. You will notice that the taste of the food you often cook far exceeds the taste of what is served at a restaurant. Start cooking for yourself today, and you will lose weight.

Trying to lose weight can be very hard if you don't diet properly, especially when you try to do so while having a fast-paced lifestyle. If you are struggling with losing weight on your own, keep in mind that there is still much that you can do to achieve such a goal. By following some tips and tricks, you can help increase your success and confidence.

Meal planning is a great way to keep yourself from overeating when you don't have time to prepare. As long as you understand the idea of portion control, it will become easier for you to make a healthy meal that doesn't leave you feeling hungry for the rest of the day.

Although that is not always possible, there are many steps you can take to achieve your weight loss goals. You can talk to your doctor, nutritionist, or personal trainer to help you find the right weight loss plan for you. You can lose weight without dieting or going to the gym by taking care of yourself. Do things good for your health, such as exercising regularly and eating a well-balanced diet. If you stay away from foods that are bad for you and maintain a healthy lifestyle, you will be healthier in the long term and easier to maintain your weight loss goals.

GLOSSARY

Adipose tissue - Commonly known as body fat. It can be found in every part of the body. It's found beneath the skin (subcutaneous fat), around internal organs (visceral fat), between muscles, in bone marrow, and in breast tissue.

Antioxidants - Molecules in your body that fight free radicals

BMI - Body Mass Index

Cirrhosis - A liver disease characterized by cell degeneration, inflammation, and fibrous tissue thickening. It's usually caused by alcoholism or hepatitis.

DNA - Deoxyribonucleic Acid

Fibromyalgia - A condition that causes pain all over the body (also known as widespread pain), as well as sleep issues, fatigue, and emotional and mental distress.

g - Grams

Hydrogenated Fats - Fatty acids that have undergone chemical modification Hydrogenated fats were oils that had their chemical structures changed to make solid fats.

Ketogenic Diet - A ketogenic diet consists of a high-fat, low-carbohydrate (sugar) diet that causes the body to break down fat into molecules known as ketones.

lb - Pounds

Lean meats - Meats with low fat content are known as lean meats. Lean meat includes skinless chicken and turkey and red meat with the fat removed, such as pork chops.

mg - milligram

Omega 3 - Omega-3 fatty acids are nutrients obtained from food (or supplements) that aid in the development and maintenance of a healthy body. They're essential for the structure of every cell wall. They also serve as an energy source and aid in the proper functioning of your heart, lungs, blood vessels, and immune system.

Omega 6 - Polyunsaturated fatty acids are found in vegetable oils, nuts, beans, seeds, and grains, with the first double bond in the hydrocarbon chain occurring between the sixth and seventh carbon atoms from the end of the molecule farthest from the carboxylic acid group.

pH - a graph that depicts the acidity or alkalinity of a solution on a logarithmic scale, with 7 representing neutral, lower values indicating more acidity, and higher values indicating more alkalinity.

RNA - Ribonucleic acid

Superfoods - a nutrient-dense food that is thought to be especially good for one's health and well-being.

Triglycerides - Glycerol and three fatty acid groups are combined to form an ester. Triglycerides are the primary components of natural fats and oils, and high blood levels indicate a higher risk of stroke.

tsp - Teaspoon

tsbp - Tablespoon

Yogi - a person who knows how to do yoga.

BIBLIOGRAPHY

https://www.bbc.co.uk/bitesize/guides/z3shycw/revision/3

https://www.nhlbi.nih.gov/education/dash-eating-plan

http://www.nasonline.org/

https://www.benefiber.com/fiber-in-your-life/daily-fiber-intake/top-10-high-fiber-foods/

https://www.webmd.com/vitamins-and-supplements/vitamins-minerals-how-much-should-you-take

https://www.cdc.gov/nchs/fastats/food-consumption.htm

http://needyourdaily.com/

http://www.healthline.com/health-topics/nutrition

https://www.webmd.com/diet/ss/slideshow-healthy-diet-tips?page=2

https://www.medicalnewstoday.com/articles/weight-loss-meal-plan#7-day-meal-plan

https://blog.myfitnesspal.com/ask-the-dietitian-whats-the-best-carb-protein-and-fat-breakdown-for-weight-loss/

https://www.healthline.com/health/yoga-for-weight-loss#sample-workout

Alkalize or Die by Dr. Theodore A. Baroody, PhD (Health Recovery Center: 1991:) (also called Alkalize or Die, an Introduction to the Diet that Could Save your Life)

Beginnings: A Fresh Way of Eating by Brenda Davis, RD and Vesanto Melina, MS, RD (Whitecap Books: 1999)

The Blender Girl Smoothies by Tess Masters (Sterling Publishing Co., Inc.: 2013)

http://source.sas.upenn.edu/flash/adn/article.cfm?id=546 Prevalence and Outcomes of Obesity in Adults

Virta Health Website https://virtahealth.com/cholesterol-lowering-dietary-approaches/

https://www.ndtv.com/food/top-10-superfoods-for-weight-loss-you-must-include-in-your-diet-1842166

www.bmiinfo.net/bmi-calculator/

https://www.healthline.com/nutrition/weight-loss-mistakes#TOC_TITLE_HDR_3

https://healthbeet.org/printable-list-for-calories-in-vegetables/

https://www.fda.gov/food/new-nutrition-facts-label/how-understand-and-use-nutrition-facts-label#:~:text=The%20Daily%20Values%20are%20reference,or%20low%20in%20a%20nutrient.

https://www.healthline.com/nutrition/1500-calorie-diet#foods-to-eat

https://medlineplus.gov/ency/patientinstructions/000892.htm

Ron Brown, The body fat guide (1997)

https://www.medicalnewstoday.com/articles/calorie-deficit#summary

https://drchatterjee.com/feel-great-lose-weight/

https://alwaysgreater.com/lose-weight-feel-good-unexpected-tip/

https://www.diabetes.co.uk/food/lean-meat.html

https://www.sciencedirect.com/topics/neuroscience/body-mass-index

www.ingramcontent.com/pod-product-compliance
Lightning Source LLC
Chambersburg PA
CBHW020037120526
44589CB00032B/418